Praise for *The Ultimate* *Male Sexual Health*

"Finally, an easy and practical approach to male sexuality. *The Ultimate Guide to Male Sexual Health* is the book that every man (and woman) will go to when questions arise about the performer and the act of the performance."

> —David Y. Josephson, MD, Program Director, Urologic Oncology and Robotic Surgery Fellowship, City of Hope National Medical Center

"Dr. Danoff, a world-class urologist, has written a world-class book that should be read by every man and woman who enjoys sex."

> —Wolfgang Puck, restaurateur and world-famous chef, Spago

"A great book. *The Ultimate Guide to Male Sexual Health* is a must-read for all men and women who love sex!"

> —Mancow Muller, host, *Mancow Experience*, WABC Talk Radio

"Dr. Danoff brings forward his deep knowledge and experience as a leading urologist in an educational and entertaining book that should address every question that most men utter only inside the confines of their doctors' exam rooms. I should tell you that their wives and girlfriends ask me the same questions, and this book is a great resource for them as well."

> —Sharron L. Mee, MD, female urologist

"A must-read for all men who care about their physical and sexual health."

> —Joe Weider, world-famous bodybuilder, fitness guru, and publisher of *Men's Fitness*

"A stimulating and educational medical guide that will renew men's lives in the bedroom and keep them out of the operating room."

> —Stuart Holden, MD, Medical Director, Prostate Cancer Foundation

"Insightful, educational, and liberating—this book is going to help a lot of people."

—Bill Paxton

"Simply the most empowering book of the millennium—a mastery of storytelling."

—Christopher S. Ng, MD, Chief, Division of Urology, Cedars-Sinai Medical Center

"At last it is great to see a volume that produces such a constant flow of information. The information fills nearly every void on the subject and finally exposes the long and short of it."

—Johnny Mathis

"One of the best books I have ever read on male sexual health; extremely well written, easy to understand, informative, and lighthearted."

—George DeJohn, host, *Train Station Fitness Show*, SportsRadio, and creator, 21 Day Body Makeover

"Where was this book when I was growing up? I could have been Superman instead of Caspar Milquetoast!"

—Terence Kingsley-Smith, writer

"*The Ultimate Guide to Male Sexual Health* is definitely original. It's also clever, informative, and entertaining."

—Ron Clark, playwright

"A book loaded with wisdom and wit, masterfully written by Dr. Dudley Seth Danoff. I recommend this book highly as a happy Dr. Danoff patient. For over thirty-five years, he has kept my 'below the belt' confidence high and my PSA low."

—Jerry Mayer, playwright and television writer and producer

The Ultimate Guide to Male Sexual Health

Also by the author

Superpotency: How to Get It, Use It, and Maintain It for a Lifetime

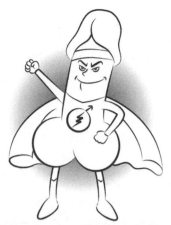

The Ultimate Guide to Male Sexual Health

How to Stay Vital at Any Age

Dudley Seth Danoff, MD, FACS

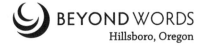

BEYOND WORDS

Hillsboro, Oregon

BEYOND WORDS

20827 N.W. Cornell Road, Suite 500
Hillsboro, Oregon 97124-9808
503-531-8700 / 503-531-8773 fax
www.beyondword.com

First Beyond Words trade paperback edition August 2017

Beyond Words Publishing is an imprint of Simon & Schuster, Inc., and the Beyond Words logo is a registered trademark of Beyond Words Publishing, Inc.

For information about special discounts for bulk purchases, please contact Beyond Words Special Sales at 503-531-8700, or specialsales@beyondword.com.

Manufactured in the United States of America

10 9 8 7 6 5 4 3 2 1

Library of Congress Control Number: 2017937560

ISBN: 978-1-58270-659-7

The corporate mission of Beyond Words Publishing, Inc.: *Inspire to Integrity*

Medical Disclaimer
The information contained in this book is intended for educational purposes only and is not intended for the treatment or prevention of disease or as a substitute for medical treatment or as an alternative to medical advice. Should you have any healthcare-related questions or concerns, please contact your physician or other qualified healthcare provider promptly.

Every attempt has been made to present accurate and timely information. The author and publisher assume neither liability nor responsibility to any person or entity with respect to any direct or indirect loss or damage caused, or alleged to be caused, by the information contained herein, or for errors, omissions, inaccuracies, or any other inconsistency within these pages, or for unintentional slights against people or organizations. The author and publisher are not associated with any manufacturers of the products mentioned and are not guaranteeing the safety of these products.

While the publisher and author have used their best efforts in preparing this book, they make no representations or warranties with respect to the accuracy or completeness of the contents of this book and specifically disclaim any implied warranties for a particular purpose. The advice and strategies contained herein may not be suitable for your situation. You should consult with a professional where appropriate. Neither the publisher nor the author shall be liable for any loss of profit or any other commercial damages, including but not limited to special, incidental, consequential, or other damages. The information in this reference is not intended to substitute for expert medical advice or treatment. It is designed to help you make informed choices. Because each individual is unique, a physician or other qualified healthcare provider must diagnose conditions and supervise treatments for each individual health problem. If an individual is under the care of a doctor or other qualified healthcare practitioner or provider and receives advice contrary to information provided in this reference, the doctor or other qualified healthcare practitioner's advice should be followed, as it is based on the unique characteristics of that individual.

To my father—a man of true penis power—often wrong
but never in doubt

Contents

Preface to the Second Edition   xi

Part 1 Everything You Need to Know about the Penis

Chapter 1: Maximizing Your Penis Power   3
    Men Are Penis Oriented   4
    We Are Tragically Ill Informed about the Penis   6
    An Epidemic of Penis Weakness   8
    Why Are We Having This Epidemic Now?   11
    A Wake-Up Call   15
    The Secret of Penis Power   16

Chapter 2: The Truth about Penis Size   19
    Looks Are Not Everything   20
    One Size Fits All   21
    Your Penis Is Not Too Small   22
    Penis Power Is Not Related to Penis Size   23
    You Are as Big as You Think You Are   25
    The Big Myth: Penile Enhancement, Phalloplasty,
        and Penile Enlargement   26

Chapter 3: Erection and Ejaculation   29
    Erections: Whatever Turns You On   30
    Tumescence: Stand Up and Be Counted   32
    Orgasms: Come Again?   33
    Semen: From Whence It Comes   34
    The Point of No Return   35
    The Refractory Period: I Want to Be Alone   37

Chapter 4: Medical Conditions That Affect Penis Power   39
    Impotence: "My Friend Has This Problem . . ."   40
    The Nerve of It: Neurological Disorders   45
    When It Cannot Go with the Flow: Vascular Disorders   45
    A Little Prick for a Big Reward: Injectable Drugs   47
    When Something Is Not Quite Right: Hormonal Disorders   47

Steroids: Big Biceps and Tiny Testes   49
Do Not Be Sicker Than You Really Are   49
Prescription Medications: Is the Pharmacist Really Your
    Enemy?   51
It's Not All Fun and Games: Recreational Drugs   53
Premature Ejaculation   55
If You Need Help, Come and Get It   56
Off the Record   58
A History of Treating PE   59

Chapter 5: Prostatic and Other Urologic Diseases   61
BPH: Don't Panic!   61
Alternatives to a Prostatectomy   63
Turn Up the Heat: TUMT   64
Call the Roto-Rooter Man   65
Prostate Cancer   66
Testicular Cancer   71
Kidney Transplants   71
The Good News   72

Chapter 6: Blue Pills and Other Medical Cures for Erectile
Dysfunction   73
Blue Magic: The Saga of "the Pills" for Men   73
It's Not Candy   74
Use with Caution   75
You Are Not Alone   76
Do Not Let the Hype Fool You   78
From Pills to Pellets: The Muse System   79
Shooting It Up: Injectable Medication   80
Surgical Procedures   83
Pump It Up: Implants   84
For the Right Reasons   86
For the Wrong Reasons   86
Mechanical Devices   87
Aphrodisiacs and Other Substances   88

Chapter 7: Performance Anxiety: When It's All in Your Head   91
Accentuate the Positive   93
Even the Strong Are Let Down Sometimes   94

Lighten Up, Dude   96
Don't Worry, Be Superpotent   99
Depression Depresses the Penis   101
Mind Games   102
Fears   103

Chapter 8: Extenuating Circumstances: When Sex
Becomes a Chore   105
The Hard Dick Syndrome   107
Hard on Demand   109
Be Careful!   110
"Blow" Is Not an Accurate Description   111
A Time and Place for Everything   112
The Sweet Smell of Success   113
The Most Unpleasant Aspect of Sex   114
Intimate Intimidation   115
When the Problem Is in Your Heart   117

Chapter 9: As Old as You Feel: The Life Story of the Penis   121
Penis Passages   123
The Early Years   124
Is It Ageless?   125
When the Going Gets Tough: Male Menopause and TRT   127
Who Needs Testosterone Replacement?   128
The Risks of TRT: Good News, but at a Price   128
Young at Heart, Young in Person   130
Andropause versus Menopause   131
Penis Posterity   132
Sex in the New Millennium   133

Chapter 10: Sexually Transmitted Diseases   135
Chlamydia: Silent but Troublesome   135
Gonorrhea: This Clap Is Not a Cheer   136
Syphilis: Next to AIDS, the Worst of All   137
Genital Herpes: Not the Scourge of the Twenty-First
Century   138
Be Alert—It's Everywhere and It's Elusive   138
AIDS: The Scourge of the Twenty-First Century   139

Chapter 11: What Women Need to Know   141
   Ladies and Gentlemen: It Begins with Communication   142
   Women's Top Ten Complaints   143
   Penis-Oriented Women Have More Fun   148

Chapter 12: Penis FAQs   149

Part 2 Becoming a Superpotent Man

Chapter 13: What's Your Penis Personality?   167
   Positive Penis Personalities   169
   Negative Penis Personalities   172

Chapter 14: What Is a Superpotent Man?   177
   Discovering Penis Power   177
   The Character of the Superpotent Man   179
   The Superpotent Man and Sex   181
   Penis Power Is Defined by Who You Are and How You
      Control Your Life   188

Chapter 15: How to Become a Superpotent Man   191
   Educate Yourself   191
   Good Health Equals Good Penis Power   193
   Penis Power Exercises   196
   Maybe Elvis Was on to Something: Pelvic Control   196
   The Harder They Come: Controlling Your Timing   198
   The "Taint" Exercises   200
   Techniques for Delaying Ejaculation   201
   Eliminate Negativity and Self-Doubt   203
   Do Not View Sex as a Performance   204
   Make Friends with Your Penis   204
   A Final Word to Women   205
   A Final Word to Men   205

Acknowledgments   207

Notes   209

Index   213

About the Author   231

Preface to the Second Edition

The seed for the creation of this book was planted in 1993 when a favorite patient of mine arrived at my office and not only suggested I write a populist book about male sexual health but held up a three-by-five card with his recommended title: *Penis Power*. This was years before the Internet, before Howard Stern, before the often-mocked ad tag line, "If your erection lasts longer than four hours, call your doctor." (Heck, if my erection lasted longer than four hours, I would call everyone I know!)

At that time, to have the word *penis* on the cover of a mainstream men's health book written by an Ivy League–educated, board-certified urologic surgeon just did not fly. The publisher of my first book (1993) insisted that the title be changed to *Superpotency*, which I thought was weak at best. I pleaded in vain. I pointed out that the word *penis* is not pejorative. It accurately describes a body part, and that word is to the urologist what the word *heart* is to the cardiologist. I shouted, "Get over it!" to no avail.

Did our puritanical forefathers instill a debilitating and often paralyzing sense of modesty in many of us? What makes so many of us giggle or blush when the word *penis* is written or spoken? There is no logic connected to this bold fact, and that has propelled me as a writer, lecturer, and teacher for the past twenty-five years to get the penis out of the closet and into the mainstream. In many ways, I have succeeded.

I have been a practicing urologic surgeon for more than forty years, and my professional goal has been to cure what I call penis weakness. I had observed that a disturbingly large number of men around the world were afflicted. It struck me that as much as the stigma of penis weakness was plaguing men in modern times, it had probably been plaguing men throughout all of history, and I began to speak out and write about the principal characteristics of this pandemic. I discovered that the vast majority of males have suffered from physical or psychological penis weakness (or both) at some point in their lives.

In most cases, the debilitating effects are compounded by a lack of knowledge by both men and women. Men who have suffered from the self-doubt and anxiety caused by penis weakness have done so with shockingly little support from the medical community.

Since those early observations, I have written extensively about how to overcome the medical and psychological factors that lead to penis weakness. My work has been read by men and women, straight couples, gay couples, and everyone in between. The overwhelming response was that the information contained in my books was vital and generated a sense of sexual enlightenment. Those individual couples who used the knowledge they gleaned from my writing developed the skills and the confidence to address the problems surrounding male genital health and sexual potency. The important information about the male sexual health that I set out to share had become the cornerstone for a new phase of the sexual revolution.

Fast forward to 2017.

With the commercial success of major pharmaceutical drugs designed to aid erectile dysfunction and their international advertising campaigns, some of the significant issues in male genital health have become part of the general social consciousness. Still, penis weakness is rampant around the world. As a physician and a husband, I am saddened to see how many men and their partners deprive themselves of the complete sexual satisfaction and enjoyment they deserve. Insecurity and uncertainty about sexual performance are the top problems for my patients, most of whom are uninformed about the nature of their penises and their bodies in general. They are also frighteningly misinformed about the medical resources available today.

In my professional lifetime, I have seen more than two hundred thousand patient penises. While each is unique, all are also remarkably alike anatomically. More important, there is enormous variation in *how* each functions in its sexual capacity. The differences in functional ability and capacity have little to do with the anatomy of a particular penis or even with a man's physical size, looks, or level of success. Mainly, they have to do with how men *perceive* their own penises. Every man must not only learn the penis's biological functions but understand that it is much more than the condition of its blood vessels and nerves—it is an organ of expression.

Penis power is a transformative concept based on positive thinking. Applying the power of positive thought to your penis can change your entire life. Your penis is what you *think* it is.

This is the basic message of *The Ultimate Guide to Male Sexual Health*. Although one of my objectives is to educate the public, this is not a medical textbook. Nothing in these pages is overly technical. And this is not a psychology book. Plenty of writers have given us treatises on the treatment of sexual dysfunction. My purpose is more practical. I am concerned with average men, men who are misinformed or confused about their penises, and extraordinary men who think they know everything but still have a lot to learn. This book is concerned with the attitudes and beliefs of men as sexual beings and the direct relationship between their personal attitudes and their penis attitudes.

Although *The Ultimate Guide to Male Sexual Health* is not a sexual manual either, you will find many practical tips, including exercises and lifestyle changes for improving penis power, sexual control, and confidence, and instructions on how to achieve a healthy, happy, and active sex life.

I want all my readers to become penis experts—to know about how the male genital system works, how and why it does not work, and how to get it to work again for as long as possible. Ultimately, I want every man to understand that no matter what his personal problems may be, as long as he makes the effort to learn how to fully express his sexual potential, he will overcome physical and psychological barriers. He will become a superpotent man, a man with penis power.

Although this book is about male sexuality and male physiology, I imagined myself speaking to both male and female readers, heterosexuals and homosexuals. The information often is blind to gender and sexual orientation. The principles presented apply to wives, husbands, girlfriends, boyfriends, or partners. Because it is awkward to keep writing "he or she" every time I refer to a man's partner, I have alternated pronouns: sometimes the partner in an example is male, sometimes female. As you read, think of your own partner and insert the appropriate pronoun.

A lot of information in these pages will surprise you. Some of it might shock or outrage you. I firmly stand behind my observations with one purpose only: to end the plague of penis weakness and the attendant cynicism, despair, and frustration that prevent the sexual happiness that all men and women deserve. Harnessing penis power to achieve superpotency is the natural birthright of every man. Its full exercise will render our lives more vigorous, healthier, and more enjoyable in every respect. A simple shift in attitude and an adjustment in your behavior patterns can give you the strength and confidence you need to achieve happiness in your sex life and ultimately in every aspect of who you are as a human being.

The Ultimate Guide to Male Sexual Health will elevate the mind, the heart, and the spirit—not just the penis. The man who has penis power is blessed, and so is the partner with whom he shares it.

Dudley Seth Danoff, MD, FACS

Part 1

Everything You Need to Know about the Penis

Chapter 1

Maximizing Your Penis Power

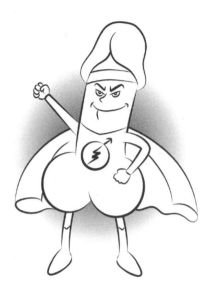

In the more than three decades that I have been practicing urology, I have treated every conceivable problem in the male genitourinary and reproductive systems—disorders ranging from minor herpes to major bladder tumors, kidney failure, and prostate cancer. I have treated men of such great wealth they could buy the hospital and men so poor they couldn't even purchase aspirin. I have treated world-famous celebrities and the people who shine their shoes, geniuses and dunces, PhDs and dropouts, men who read voraciously and men who cannot read a word. I have treated the young, middle-aged, and elderly: heterosexuals, homosexuals, bisexuals, transsexuals, and nonsexuals; and married, single, divorced, and widowed men. I have evaluated the promiscuous, the monogamous, and the celibate. All this experience has taught me that, despite the vast differences among them, all men have certain things in common:

- Men are penis oriented. In the minds of men, the penis reigns supreme.

- Most men (and almost all women) are woefully ignorant about the male sexual apparatus.
- An alarming percentage of men are plagued by penis weakness or penis insecurity.

Men Are Penis Oriented

Penis oriented means that a man's personality, behavior, and outlook on life are governed in large part by his image of his penis. The biological and emotional signals sent to a man by his penis make him "penocentric." Usually, this idea has pejorative connotations, but I don't mean *penocentric* pejoratively. I am asserting as a fact the dominance of the penis over a man's being: his self-image, attitude, and behavior. There are extremes—the Don Juans, Casanovas, exhibitionists, and men who are obsessed with sex—but what most people don't understand is that all men are penis oriented. This is simply the way nature intended men to be.

In many respects, the penis is the organ of a man's essence, the axis around which the male body and personality rotate. This observation is obvious in our rich heritage of bawdy humor. Is any body part the subject of more jokes than the penis? You may know the famous joke about a man who says to his girlfriend, "Women don't have any brains," to which she replies, "That's because we don't have penises to put them in," or the riddle a female patient once posed to me: What do you call the superfluous skin around the penis? Answer: A man. What about the young son and daughter taking a bath together? The daughter asks her mother if that "thing" between her brother's legs is his brain, and the mother replies, "Not yet!"

Consider the vast number of nicknames assigned to the penis. A partial list of terms I've heard in my life and in my practice includes *apparatus, appendage, bat, battering ram, bone, bone piccolo, cock, dick, dingaling, dong, engine, equipment, gadget, gladius* (a Latin word meaning "sword"; the Latin word *vagina* means "sheath"), *goober, hook, horn, instrument, Johnson, John Thomas, joint, Jolly Roger, machine, manhood, manroot, member, mighty one-eye, one-eyed trouser snake, organ, pecker, peenie, peepee, peter, pisser, pistol, prick, putz, rod, roger, salami, schlong, schmuck, shaft, thing, third leg, tool, wang, weapon, weewee, wick, wiener, works, yard,* and *zapper.* Individual men, and sometimes their lovers, tag their penises with affectionate nicknames. A patient's wife called his penis Helmut because its head reminded her of a helmet. A college friend called his Winchester after the rifle, but when flower power came into vogue, he dropped that in favor of Mellow Yellow. Robin Williams used to refer to Mr. Happy in his stand-up routines; Lyndon Johnson, true to form, called his Jumbo; and the King of Rock 'n' Roll referred to his favorite appendage as Little Elvis.

In a man's psyche, the penis is king, ruling its owner. Sometimes, like a potentate who follows the will of his people, the penis does a man's bidding. Other times, like a dictator, it commands by its own rules—rules that men cannot always comprehend. As a monarch, the penis acts in unpredictable, enigmatic ways—sometimes despotic, capricious, and selfish and at other times benevolent, magnanimous, and wise.

When King Penis issues a command, a man has little power to disobey. The penis can turn the mind, emotions, and senses into obedient serfs.

Understanding the powerful correlation between the dictates of the penis and men's behavior is critical. My father often said, "When it's soft, I'm hard, and when it's hard, I'm soft." What he meant was that the penis is an unpredictable creature.

Every wise woman knows the worst time to ask a man for something she wants is when he is sexually frustrated. Far better to ask when blood has rushed to his loins. His willpower has followed, and he will sell his soul for satisfaction. The best time to ask a man for anything is just after he has had a satisfying orgasm, when his essence has become as soft as his sated member.

On a more abstract level, a powerful connection exists between how men perceive their penises and how they perceive themselves. A man who likes his penis and has confidence in his organ also has trust and confidence in himself. Conversely, a man who distrusts or resents his penis and is insecure about its size or ability to perform tends to have poor self-esteem.

It is not clear which comes first, self-image or penis image. A man who is unsure of himself sexually or has embarrassing sexual experiences (such as premature ejaculation or failure to get an erection) will be shadowed in other aspects of his life by insecurity and self-doubt. A man whose self-regard takes a blow in his professional life may carry that negative feeling into the bedroom. This dynamic can also work in a positive way. If a man satisfies himself and his partner in the evening, he will probably approach his work with self-assurance in the morning; if he comes home from the *board*room with the esteem of his colleagues and the memory of a job well done, he is much more likely to glide boldly and energetically into the *bed*room.

The penis is an extension of the ego and at the same time shapes the ego. The penis receives its marching orders from the brain and at the same time dictates to the brain. Sexuality is an essential part of everyone's life, a fundamental human drive second only to basic survival. This truth of human existence deserves open discussion. Instead we often either deny it or act as if it were a curse inflicted by the devil. We should celebrate sexuality as one of our most valuable gifts.

We Are Tragically Ill Informed about the Penis

In this age of the Internet when pornographic pictures are easier to find than photographs of world leaders, and seminude bodies can be seen gyrating on prime-time television, the penis remains closeted. Thanks to the candor of the women's movement and the social importance of childbearing, men and women are relatively well informed about women's sexuality and the anatomy of the female reproductive system. But when it comes to the penis and its attendant components, both sexes are plagued by ignorance. An awareness of the real issues surrounding the penis and male sexuality has in recent years been triggered by the increase in public advertisement of such male sexual enhancement products as Viagra, Levitra, and Cialis, but I am always amazed by how underinformed and misinformed my patients are about their own penises. The myths I hear about the penis are mind boggling.

Misinformation and lack of information are everywhere. In classrooms teachers mention the penis only in attenuated descriptions of how conception takes place. Most fathers are not much help either. They have "the talk" with their sons only when forced and often rush through it as if they cannot wait to change the subject. These brief conversations are usually relegated to a form of the old *Hill Street Blues* tagline, "Be careful out there," or my favorite old saw, "Son, you're playing with a loaded gun now!"

Doctors offer little help. Pediatricians discuss the penis with adolescents only if they observe a physical abnormality or when they provide warnings about pregnancy or sexually transmitted diseases. Nowhere do young men learn the biological facts—or about the mental and emotional connection that exists between themselves and their penises. And as men get older, doctors talk about the penis only when a patient brings up a problem. Even in general physical examinations, physicians take at most a cursory look at the genitals for signs of gross abnormalities. With older men, doctors might perform the requisite examination of the prostate gland and provide a questionnaire to ask if a patient is having problems with his sex drive, usually coupled with an offer to buy an erectile dysfunction medication—an approach hardly offering an opening for beneficial discussion.

Often the very word *penis* still has a peculiar shock value, inciting a giggle and a blush. The word puts many men on guard, even in a doctor's office. Physicians often are undereducated in the area of men's sexual health, learning only the basic anatomy and the biological details of what takes place when the penis performs its various functions, and doctors and patients alike learn little about the *penis mystique*, that curious realm where the hard data of biology meets the unpredictable and mysterious realm of the mind and emotions.

Doctors should be able to competently answer these questions:
- What makes the penis work and what makes it *not* work?
- Why does the penis seem to have a mind of its own?
- Why does the penis get hard sometimes and not others?

- Why are some sexual experiences more satisfying than others, even though the exact same reflex action occurs with every orgasm?
- What is normal and what is not?

Men wonder about all these topics but often are too embarrassed to ask, and if they do ask, they usually get inadequate answers. The truth is that we do not know enough about these issues scientifically, and the psychic realm of the penis is being ignored in medical education, except in psychiatry classes where discussions are most often confined to abnormalities. If men cannot turn to doctors for this vital information, whom can they ask? Unfortunately, most men get their penis education from locker-room banter, pornography, racy novels, and the mass media. This is not education. Knowledge of the penis is so central to a man's being—so natural, so normal, and so vital—we must bring it out of the closet and into the light of day.

An Epidemic of Penis Weakness

Penis weakness is one of the best-kept secrets in America and probably throughout the world. If my experience as a busy urologist is an accurate gauge, the last twenty years have seen a dramatic rise in both real sexual dysfunction and imagined inadequacy. Far more of the imagined variety exists: huge numbers of men *think* they are deficient in some way or *assume* something is wrong with them or *fear* they are abnormal. Some come to see me specifically to talk about their sexual concerns, though most are driven by kidney or bladder disorders or prostate conditions and eventually find a way to bring up their penis anxieties.

A patient might have a minor complaint about a blemish, an irritation, an itch, or a burning sensation when he urinates, but he almost always has something else on his mind. I can almost predict the moment—as he is putting on his pants or reaching for the exam room doorknob—when he says, "By the way, Doc . . . " and then expresses one of two concerns—size or performance. With all due respect to Dr. Freud, women do not have penis envy; they have penis *curiosity*. It is *men* who have penis envy. "Is it of normal size, Doc? Shouldn't it be bigger?" Some even ask if I have a way to make it longer or wider. More frequently questions are about performance in one of three areas: sex drive, erections, and ejaculation.

Older men worry because they seem to have lost their libidos.

Middle-aged men are upset because they used to desire sex as often as they could get it, but now they want to make love only a few times a month.

Even young men are occasionally concerned: "My friends are horny all the time. Sex is all they think about. I'm not the same. Is there something wrong with me?"

Men's erection worries include "I can't get one"; "It takes me a long time to get hard"; "I can't get it up more than once a night now"; and "I lost it right in the middle of foreplay!" Ejaculation distress includes "I can't come anymore"; "I used to have a big payload, and now it's just a little squirt"; and "My partner complains it takes me forever." And the biggest panic-inducer of all is, "My lover says I come too fast."

A small percentage of sexual dysfunction complaints indicate bona fide medical problems, usually in older men with organic disorders that impede their ability to achieve an erection adequate for penetration (the classic definition of impotence). A number of physiological conditions can cause impotence, including arteriosclerosis, diabetes, hormonal disorders, injuries, multiple sclerosis, reactions to medication, substance abuse, and the physical effects of aging. Physicians have made tremendous advances in the science of diagnosis and treatment of erectile dysfunction, and sophisticated tests can now determine the exact cause of the problem or, equally important, can rule out underlying medical causes.

Wherever there is even a remote possibility of a medical condition, I treat the situation as such. However, only a small number of patients who complain about their penises have genuine medical conditions, while the majority of complaints I hear are expressions of insecurity with no medical basis, variations on fundamental anxieties: "Am I normal, Doc? Am I okay?"

In most cases, my answer is unequivocally yes.

I tell my patients that penis power is 1 percent between the legs and 99 percent between the ears. This, of course, is a figure of speech more than a real statistic, but I stand by the spirit of my words—the majority of men have perfectly normal apparatuses, and whatever problem they have, or *think* they have, originates in their minds. This is the case even if the problem expresses itself in a penis that refuses to obey orders.

Some men have chronic sexual dysfunction that is cause for serious concern, dysfunction that affects not only their personal satisfaction and their self-image but also their relationships and the happiness of their partners. When these problems are rooted in deep psychological conditions due to depression, childhood sexual abuse, or debilitating inner conflict, they are best served by a qualified psychiatrist or psychotherapist.

Such cases, however, are exceptions. Most men can help themselves with a simple change of behavior and an attitude adjustment. The majority of men who worry about their penises are perturbed because of the erroneous notion that they don't measure up to some (mythological) standard.

Self-doubt is the biggest enemy of the penis! The nature of the brain-penis axis is so delicate that a lack of confidence or a fear of failure can easily create a self-fulfilling prophecy. If you *think* you are abnormal, if you are anxious about performing adequately, if you are afraid that your partner might be disappointed, chances are you have already worried yourself into creating the very problems you fear.

This is the vicious cycle: doubt leads to penis weakness, a bad experience increases self-doubt, and during the next sexual encounter, the anxiety level is even higher, making the chances of the problem repeating itself greater.

Most men who complain of penis problems are either perfectly normal and don't realize it or inflate their own difficulties by allowing themselves to get sucked into the quicksand of doubt. An injection of simple education and a strong dose of reassurance is astonishingly effective at curing these types of penis problems.

Why Are We Having This Epidemic Now?

I have witnessed an increased development of penis weakness over the last thirty years, with powerful social and historical factors contributing to and continuing to create penis weakness. One factor is increased stress. Men today work long hours without enough sleep, exercise, or relaxation and often are psychologically drained and physically exhausted when they get home from work. Add financial anxiety; societal pressure; traffic jams; and conflicts with bosses, coworkers, clients, spouses, and children—all elements that are not conducive either to maximum sexual performance or maximum happiness!

Compound this with the media's romanticized image of marriage and family life, and impossible expectations are created. Being at your best at anything, especially sex, is difficult when you feel out of sorts physically or your mind is somewhere else, preoccupied by other problems. Stress, tension, and anxiety exact a heavy toll on any intimate relationship, polluting the atmosphere and filling the bedroom with emotional toxins. Stress also has definite medical consequences that work against normal sexual function. During the stress response, blood moves away from the genitals to supply the large muscle groups of the arms and legs. Anxiety, including performance anxiety, can increase the activity of the sympathetic nervous system, boosting the flow of norepinephrine, a chemical that constricts blood vessels. This condition is precisely the opposite of what is necessary for an erection—a smooth flow of blood to the penis through open vascular channels.

The drugging of the American male is another major factor in the decline of penis power. The use of alcohol and drugs in an attempt to cope with stress will only compound the problem. As Shakespeare wisely observed, alcohol "provokes the desire, but it takes away the performance."[1] The same is true of drugs, including nicotine and prescription medications. The craze over "Vitamin V" (Viagra) is hardly the solution.

To men who suffer from penis weakness, the women's movement, for all its welcome advances, has also contributed to the problem. With increased awareness of female sexuality and female orgasm and the generally open discussion of women's sexual needs, men have the added pressure of having to know the intricate secrecies of female sexuality with an expectation that they will perform with the expertise of a twenty-four-year-old pornography star. For some men, this might not be a problem, but for most, sex is an obstacle course—a track filled with snares and hurdles in which one scores points for technique as well as for reaching the finish line and satisfying one's partner. Many men believe they have a responsibility not just to bring a woman to orgasm but to multiple, ecstatic, earth-shattering orgasms. Now that's pressure!

Both men and women expect sexual satisfaction, and partners have a responsibility to work together through communication and understanding to achieve mutual satisfaction. Every man should cater to his partner's pleasure if for no other reason than to enhance his own. It is important to acknowledge that men and women have been insensitive to the high level of performance anxiety brought on by the new rules, a situation made even more complicated by the enormous range of variation in female sexuality.

The widespread use of vibrators and other sensual aids has further complicated matters for men. I have had female patients whose use of vibrators has irritated their urinary tracts, but when I ask why they continue to use them, they often reply that the vibrator gives them a level of sexual excitement they never obtain with their husbands or boyfriends. Some patients have become so dependent on their vibrators they have stopped having sex altogether. While no vibrator has lips, hands, or a tongue, nor can one be programmed to hug you when you need to be hugged, no human penis can measure up to an inanimate object that is always hard, is always ready to go, never asks for anything in return, and can be totally controlled.

While this might be a minor factor in male insecurity today, the vibrator problem must not be overlooked. My hope is that men will read this book and elevate their sexuality to a level of superpotency, that vibrators will no longer compete with and replace the actual organ they attempt to replicate.

The main reason for the increase in penis weakness is the way in which men learn about sex. Some confusion is due to a simple lack of accurate information. A teenage patient asked me about a minor abrasion on his penis, and as I examined him and prescribed a medication, I could tell that he wanted to say something more. He finally found the courage to tell me that he had sex with a girl the previous weekend and could not ejaculate. He was terrified that something was wrong with him. I asked about his prior sexual experience, and after he got over his initial awkwardness with me, he admitted that he had treated himself to a veritable orgy of masturbation on the day of his embarrassing experience. I explained that anyone who ejaculates six times in an afternoon might have trouble doing it again two hours later. He was so relieved to hear this, I thought he would kiss me.

Had this young man never asked, he might have carried the false feeling of inadequacy into subsequent sexual encounters, resulting in a downward spiral of self-doubt. This happens too often to young men who do not know that lost erections and premature ejaculation are common among their peers. Because they are too self-conscious to mention the subject, they assume that something is wrong with them, and in many cases, they remain inhibited for years, if not decades.

Disappointments due to anxiety are far more likely when a young couple hops into bed without having experienced the old-fashioned waiting period during which couples develop trust and affection. I am not advocating old conventions. Casual sex can be terrific when people are knowledgeable, careful, and self-assured. But when participants are nervous, awkward, and unfamiliar with each other, sex can be traumatic, and a few early traumas can scar a young man for a long time.

The natural bravado of men supersedes their need for accurate information. Teenagers in the locker room or school cafeteria are not likely to hear confessions like, "Hey, guys, I was making out with Suzie last weekend, and I came in my pants before I even had her blouse off," or "Man, I was just about to do the deed when my dick folded up like an umbrella." Incidents like these occur every weekend all over the world, but even best friends seldom confess such humiliations to each other. What an adolescent boy *is* likely to hear are wildly exaggerated or completely imaginary tales of sexual exploits, which become the standards by which he will then measure himself.

The same kind of macho posturing that is found in malls and on schoolyards also exists on golf courses and in bars, factories, and offices, so the widespread myth that a "real man" is ready to get it on any time and any place and knows everything there is to know about sex and women persists well into adulthood. Such a man never doubts his virility, is never nervous or scared, and can satisfy without fail any partner who is willing. Instead of the real face of male sexuality, most men see the illusions and myths.

Self-doubt created by a lack of penis education is magnified by the mass media's obsession with sleek, young, perfectly proportioned bodies. Those handsome hunks with rippling six-packs and perfect pectoralis muscles who parade before our eyes in movies and magazines present an ideal of masculinity few men can live up to. When you look in the mirror and see something different from those media images, you think what you see in the mirror is inferior, even abnormal. That chips away at your self-esteem.

This is not just about vanity—it's about sex. These popular images represent idealized models of masculinity. Each little dent in your self-image adds to the sum of doubt that you carry with you to the bedroom. Your image of your penis, your perception of it, your attitude toward it, and therefore, your sense of yourself as a sexual being, are directly linked to the way you view your body.

Another media-related factor is the idealized image of the sex act itself. Sex is one of the few activities we do not learn about by watching other people do it—not *real* people at any rate. But we peek through the keyhole by watching pornographic films and even mainstream movies. With the aid of our imagination, we spy on couples in books. This is hardly an education in realism. If a man's primary source of sex education is pornographic movies and books, he'll have the impression that a real man is a sculpted masterpiece with a huge penis that becomes as hard as stone on a moment's notice and stays that way, throbbing and plunging and pounding, until he and his lover—who is gorgeous, perfectly proportioned, and insatiable—with the perfect timing of synchronized swimmers, have simultaneous, Richter-registering orgasms. Even with Hollywood scriptwriters, directors, set designers and special-effects wizards and the London Symphony Orchestra accompanying your tryst, you would rarely duplicate these glorified performances. When reality doesn't measure up to the imagined ideal, men often think they are failures. And the focal point of their disappointment is, of course, their penis. "What's wrong with it? Why can't it be bigger and harder? Why doesn't it do what those throbbing pistons do?"

I hear those questions almost every day. Far too many of my patients think they should have a two-foot-long shaft of solid steel between their legs that can pump and pound for hours on end.

That's not a penis. That's a Home Depot pneumatic drill from aisle six!

Most men measure themselves against standards built on fantasy and interpret normal experiences as signs of failure. Enormous variety exists among men with respect to sex drive, capacity, preferences, and satisfaction, yet most men assume there is a "normal" and worry that every little sexual idiosyncrasy they have is a sign of abnormality. Worse, if they have a disappointing or embarrassing experience, they panic, resulting in significant self-doubt, which further creates fear, anxiety, and inhibition. These feelings are bigger obstacles to sexual happiness than having a construction crew in your bedroom. They may be even bigger obstacles than having your mother-in-law there!

Every man I have ever known has, at one time or another, lost an erection or ejaculated sooner than he would have liked. Every man is, at times, not interested in sex. Every man has failed to satisfy a partner. Men who take such events in stride know that they are perfectly normal and march without hesitation to their next sexual encounter.

These are the men who have penis power.

A Wake-Up Call

Nothing is more wonderful than the uninhibited expression of sexuality. Nothing is more glorious than the joyful sharing of physical pleasure between two generous, enthusiastic human beings. The current plague of confusion and self-consciousness causes most men to have less sex than they would like and to enjoy the sex they *do* have a lot less.

Sex is life's cheapest luxury and should be fun and relaxing, a simple, natural pleasure that *erases* worries, tensions, and burdens. But for too many men and women it has become a worrisome task. Using your penis for the purpose nature intended not only is one of life's great pleasures but also is good for your health in general—for your cardiovascular health, your mood, and your psychological well-being. Penis use is a natural tranquilizer with no bad side effects. Men who are sexually frustrated tend to be tense and irritable, while men who are sexually satisfied and feel good about themselves as sexual beings tend to have a positive outlook and a warm glow of health. Sex is also excellent for overall fitness. It benefits circulation, stimulates the nervous system and the prostate gland, and clears up mental cobwebs.

Contrary to certain myths, you cannot wear out your penis with sexual activity. You do not have a preset allotment of orgasms. As the childhood ditty goes, "Use it, use it, you cannot abuse it, and if you don't, you're gonna lose it."

One word of caution: as a physician who has treated numerous AIDS and HIV patients and who has seen many of them die, I'd be the last person to advise anyone to be carefree in his sexual life, but the tragic AIDS epidemic should not inhibit responsible adults who are aware of the risks involved in various practices and who understand how to use sound judgment and the necessary means of prevention.

The Secret of Penis Power

The real secret of penis power is embodied in this simple premise:

> If you become absolutely at ease with your penis, the quality of your life will dramatically change for the better.

My goal with this book is to destroy penis weakness in all its forms—chronic or occasional, actual or imagined—to eliminate self-doubt and inhibition. In the pursuit of this goal, this book will erase the mythology surrounding the penis and empower men to enjoy every ounce of pleasure this wonderful organ was intended to give. The information provided will help men have a better understanding and greater control in their sexual and romantic relationships and will help women become experts in the nurturing and care of the penises in their lives.

Used properly, the lessons in this book will help you become super-potent. This does not mean you will have a King Kong–like erection for a week straight. Nor does it imply you will become a stereotypical stud.

I do not define superpotency according to arbitrary standards of frequency, endurance, or technique. Rather, the concept of penis power means achieving maximum enjoyment and satisfaction for both you and your partner, as determined by your own standards, desires, and tastes. *Penis power* means harnessing the full potential of your penis by treating it with all the respect and appreciation it deserves. Learning to do so will do more for your self-esteem than a year's worth of self-help workshops. It will do more for the sorry state of sexual relationships than any talk show, how-to video, or program found on television today.

My message is simple:

- Your penis is as big as you think it is; if you think big, you are big.
- Your penis behaves the way you tell it to, and you can learn how to control it.
- You are as potent as you think you are.
- You are okay, and your penis is okay.

A minority of men do have medical conditions that impede the normal sexual function of their penises. You need to be aware of the conditions that may impair a man's sexual ability, as well as other physical factors that can affect the penis, and understand that with today's medical advancements, many of these organic penile infirmities can be overcome. Unless you are one of those exceptions, you do not need specialized medical care or intensive psychotherapy. You need the basic facts you'll find in this book.

Chapter 2

The Truth about Penis Size

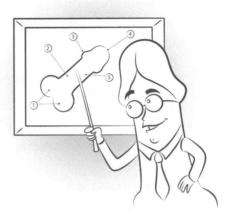

Most people have a pretty good idea how the heart works, where the lungs and kidneys are located, and what happens to food as it works its way through the digestive system. They even know how babies are born. But nearly half of the human bodies in the world have this odd-looking appendage dangling between their legs, and people know nothing about it. If it were not for that "tail" (the Latin translation of penis), you would not be reading this page! My patients, both men and women, ask so many elementary questions about the anatomy and functioning of the penis that I am often amazed.

The irony is that most people have been curious about the penis ever since they were old enough to notice that boys have one and girls do not, but for some reason, this natural curiosity is suppressed. As children, we are told that our questions about the genitals and about sex will be answered when we are "older," but most adults are too self-conscious to seek out the information.

Since you are reading this book, I commend your courage and maturity as you come to fully understand the complex and fascinating details of male anatomy and sexuality.

Looks Are Not Everything

The penis is odd looking, with wrinkles and folds and a wriggling network of red-and-blue vein pathways. Aesthetically, most people, regardless of gender, do not find the penis attractive. Some even find it ugly.

I am reminded of a conversation with the very sophisticated wife of a fellow urologist. We were talking one day about a case of hypospadias, a rare congenital abnormality in which the urinary opening (meatus) is not in its normal location at the tip of the penis but somewhere down along the shaft. This deformity is often compounded by a fibrous band of tissue known as a chordee that gives a peculiar downward curvature to the penis.

I asked her if she knew what a hypospadias was. She said, "Yes. That's a penis that's uglier than usual!"

Most women, when they talk about how handsome a man is, might praise his strong, muscular physique or giggle over his biceps, legs, or buttocks. Seldom will they single out his penis as being attractive. When women hoot and holler over male strippers at Chippendales, they are reacting to everything *but* the penis, excited by the fabulous bodies of those gyrating hunks and the way the dancers tease them with their *unexposed* penises. I wish our genitals were not overcast by a shadow of repugnance or deemed inappropriate objects of discussion or admiration. Nothing is intrinsically ugly about the penis (or the vagina, which is equally unappreciated for its perceived lack of physical beauty). Our cultural perception reflects a conservative and puritanical past with roots in traditions that hold sex—and therefore the sexual organs—to be dirty and debased.

Now is the time for the penis (and the vagina) to be viewed as a beautiful part of the body, celebrated and discussed openly. If you cannot find it in yourself to feel that way about *all* genitals, then at least see your own as a beautiful part of *your* body and try to view your partner's with the same perspective. Your attitude toward your penis reflects your general attitude toward sex and the specific way in which you relate to your genitals. Just as parents see their own children as beautiful regardless of their actual features, so too can we look at our genitals and find them lovely to behold.

Some of you may think this sounds "New Agey" or trite, but I encourage all men to seriously consider the way in which they view their own genitals. A radical change in perspective toward your penis is an integral step toward overcoming self-doubt and self-consciousness. It is equally important for women to muster up the courage and strength to overcome these backward views regarding genitals.

Why? Just as children who are told they are beautiful think more highly of themselves, a man feels better about himself—and his sexuality—if he's told his penis is beautiful. The more beauty your partner sees in your penis, the more *you* will like what you see. As a result, you will attribute more good qualities to your penis and bring more confidence into the bedroom.

If the penis were less concealed, if it were more openly portrayed in art and film, it might come to be better appreciated as an object of aesthetic pleasure. We would come to respect the vast range of differences among penises. In my thirty years in medicine, I have seen more male organs than you would see if you filled the Rose Bowl with naked men. I have never seen two that look quite alike. Greater visibility in mass media and art might demystify the penis and might make men less self-conscious about their own. That acceptance, in turn, would raise the overall level of penis power.

One Size Fits All

More than general appearance, men are concerned with size. I cannot count the number of men who have asked me if theirs was "normal." No man has ever worried that it might be too big.

This preoccupation is one of the saddest and most complicated issues I encounter. Men compensate for their insecurity with more jokes about penis *size* than anything else. One example is the joke about the man playing golf; he hits the ball into the rough. While he is looking for the ball, he happens to see a pair of tiny feet sticking out of some tangled brambles. He hears a little Irish voice calling for help, and as he pulls the little feet out from the brush, he's surprised to see he has freed a leprechaun, who, in appreciation, grants him one wish. Without any hesitation, the golfer says, "I want the biggest dick you can give me!" A moment later the man's penis becomes so long that it sticks out of the bottom of his golf pants, drags on the ground, and needs to be tucked into his socks. Overall, it becomes a nuisance. The next time out on the links, the man meets the leprechaun, who asks, "How's it hangin'?" The man explains his predicament, and the leprechaun, feeling compassionate, grants him another wish. Without hesitation, the man says, "Can you make my legs about four inches longer?"

That joke says everything you need to know about what penis size means within the minds of men. The *myth* that size—length and width—matters is one of the cruelest hoaxes ever perpetrated on mankind.

Your Penis Is Not Too Small

The variation in size among human penises is less than that among hands, fingers, or noses. Penises can be as short as one and a half inches or as long as eight inches. The number of organs that fall at the extremes is exceedingly few. The average length of a penis in its fully flaccid (relaxed, limp, normal) state is about four inches. The overwhelming majority of men fall within centimeters of that average. Penis girth varies less, ranging between one and one and a half inches in diameter when flaccid.

A very tall man might have a longer penis than a short man, just as he will probably have bigger feet and hands. The difference in penis size between two such men will be *far less* than that of their other appendages. A short man's hand might be three full inches shorter than that of a tall man. He might wear a size eight shoe compared to the taller man's size thirteen. But his penis might only be a fraction of an inch shorter. I have often seen penises on short men that were as big, or bigger, than those of most professional basketball players.

Most men are far more concerned with the size of the *erect* penis. The erect penis averages about six inches in length (although most of my patients prefer the phrase "half a foot long"). More importantly, the variation in the size of the erect penis is far less than that of the flaccid penis. If one man's penis is five inches long when soft and another's is three, that two-inch difference is likely to shrink to near zero when they become erect. The smaller penis may even be bigger when erect.

Nature wanted humans to propagate and so made it possible for almost any man, regardless of his overall size, to mate with any woman. When you hear a man brag that his penis is a foot long, take it with a few grains of salt. He is either a rare exception or a liar. He might be telling the truth if he is adding to his measurement that portion of the penis deep inside the pelvic cavity where the penis actually begins. We do not normally think about this as part of the length of the penis—it's an idea akin to measuring a hose attached to a sink inside a house.

The biggest penis I have ever seen belonged to a short, pleasant, mild-mannered, pious man in his eighties who was having prostate surgery. He had been married to the same woman his entire adult life, and neither of them had the slightest idea how relatively huge the penis that had sired their nine children was, nor did they care. Half the nurses in the building wanted to assist me just to view this magnificent organ. The point is not that men and women are not *interested* in size, but that most wives and lovers do not much care.

Penis Power Is Not Related to Penis Size

Once I assure my patients that their penises are within the normal range, I hammer home this crucial point: *superpotency has nothing to do with the size of your penis.* When a superpotent man makes love, he is immersed in the erotic physical sensations, as well as the feelings of intimacy and tenderness. The last thing on his mind, or on the mind of his lover, is the *size* of his penis.

I have seen men with larger-than-average penises who are plagued by sexual dysfunction. I have seen men with relatively small penises who represent the quintessence of superpotency.

I have never had a woman complain to me that her man's penis was too small. It is conceivable that some women make such complaints to their gynecologists or to female physicians, but in my decades of experience, a prodigious penis is simply not a priority for the vast majority of women. My female colleagues agree with me.

A much more common complaint is that a lover's penis is *too big*. Intercourse can be painful for a woman whose vagina cannot accommodate a large penis. Women have asked me if I can make their partner's penis *harder* or perhaps attach it to a more loving and sensitive guy. Women have sometimes asked about the feasibility of surgically reducing the size; never has anyone asked me to make her partner's penis longer or wider. No procedure can reduce penis size just as no legitimate and safe procedure exists to make penises bigger. Penile prostheses, which I often implant surgically to treat organic impotence, do not enlarge the penis. They merely fill the vascular compartments (corpora) in the penis with a firm, inert material that makes the penis hard enough for penetration.

The old homily "It's not how big it is, but how you use it" is one of those penis clichés that holds up to close scrutiny. Many of my women patients complain that their men do not get aroused often enough or are not imaginative enough. They complain that their penises do not get *hard* enough. One female patient of mine, a true sage, said, "I don't care how long it is. I don't care how fat it is. I don't care how good-looking it is. I just care how *hard* it is!"

Denying that some women do not have preferences for certain types of penises would be wrong, but in most relationships in which two people care enough about being with each other, they will find ways to make their sex lives work so that both parties are satisfied.

Some of the fascination with large penises can be attributed to the general cultural viewpoint that "bigger is better." The phallus is a symbol of potency, physical strength, and masculinity. Psychologically, then, it makes sense that some people conclude that bigger penises are better. The fascination with large penises is not unlike an attraction to large breasts or shapely behinds. Those features might enhance the sexual experience because they fulfill a fantasy, but physiologically and anatomically, what occurs during intercourse has nothing to do with the size of any body part. The orgasm is exactly the same regardless of the physical features of the partner. An experience that may feel different is actually a result of the power of the mind and the emotions.

Sound physiological reasons explain why size does not contribute much to satisfaction. Nature, in its wisdom, placed the principal nerve endings that produce sexual pleasure and orgasm right up front. By this grand design, they can be stimulated *regardless of size*. The man's areas are on the glans, and the woman's are on the clitoris. This means that any penis is capable of satisfying any woman. By experimenting with different positions and by using hands, lips, or even the penis to stimulate the clitoris directly, any man can secure satisfaction for his partner.

Different women are aroused in different ways. I have talked to women who complained that even though their men were endowed with large penises, they were unable to be satisfied during sex. Any sexually intimate couple must discuss their preferences and experiment with different positions. Combining penile stimulation with the simultaneous aid of hands and lips is also a great way to help bring a partner to orgasm.

At this point some of you are probably shaking your heads, convinced that penis size matters. I know what kinds of penises are out there and feel safe in saying that most of the issue with penis size is between our ears—in our minds—and not between our legs.

You Are as Big as You Think You Are

The only advantage a man with a large penis might have is that he *thinks* he has an advantage. The myth of the importance of penis size is so strong that if a man thinks he is exceptionally big, he might start *acting* big, developing such a strong sense of confidence and penis pride early in life that this alone endows him with exceptional penis power.

The fact is, though, far more men think that they are too small, and the precise opposite self-fulfilling prophecy takes place for these men. This insecurity usually starts at puberty, when boys start to be self-conscious about everything associated with masculinity. Most boys magnify any sign of inadequacy they perceive. They compare themselves to older boys or men, or to peers who happen to mature faster. They look down and see a puny, shriveled gherkin, then look across the locker room at someone else's dangling zucchini. They feel inferior. Sometimes these feelings get even worse with age. If men hang around with guys who brag—or more likely, lie—about the size of their erections or tell jokes about small penises, their insecurity may worsen. Watching pornographic movies with deceptive lighting and camera tricks heightens men's feelings of inadequacy.

Many men feel worse about size as they age because they *think* their penises are shrinking. Chubby men may appear to have small penises—especially in their own eyes—because they are looking down over a potbelly. In obese men, the shaft of the penis has to traverse two, three, or four inches of prepubic fat from under the pubic bone, where the base of the penis starts, until it is visible. Slim men may appear to have big penises. In truth difference in size is not significant, especially when the penis is erect. A man who does not learn the truth about penis size can be shadowed by a sense of inadequacy throughout his adult life. *Think small and you will be small.* Fortunately, the corollary is equally true: *think big and you will be big.* What really matters is the size of your self-esteem and the size of your heart, *not* the size of your penis, and besides, size is strictly genetically determined.

The Big Myth: Penile Enhancement, Phalloplasty, and Penile Enlargement

Every day, I get six or more e-mail offers for ways to make my penis longer, wider, thicker, or more appealing, promises to "satisfy my dreams" with a magic potion or a ridiculous surgery. As my friend Professor Thomas Lue of the University of California, San Francisco, a world-class authority on erectile dysfunction, told me, "The surgical 'enlargement' of the penis is no more effective than taking your penis and whacking it with a large wooden mallet, which essentially results in a flattened, squashed, and mangled 'Polish sausage' effect."

There is no effective way to enhance penis size. The five oral erectile dysfunction drugs currently on the market (Viagra, Cialis, Levitra, Staxyn, Stendra) give one a firmer, *but not a bigger*, penis. One "penis enlargement" surgery that has been foisted on the unsophisticated consumer consists of nothing more than cutting the suspensory ligaments of the penis. These ligaments attach to the undersurface of the pubic bone, and cutting them gives the appearance of length by allowing the penis to hang lower. Absolutely no length is gained in the erect penis.

Another technique involves applying grafted material (usually skin, fat, or a synthetic material) within the shaft of the penis. This usually leads to an unsightly deformity and can cause serious and damaging complications. Every man's penis is determined at birth by the size of the corpora cavernosa (the two chambers within the shaft of the penis that fill with blood during an erection).

Think of the corpora cavernosa as sausage casings, the size of which is predetermined by heredity. When filled with blood at the height of stimulation, both the length and the girth are fixed. Even when surgeons implant a penile prosthesis, we cannot insert a larger implant than the genetically predetermined size of the corpora can accommodate. When surgical quacks and adventurists try to stuff the corpora with autologous fat or other grafting material, the result not only is hideous but also invariably results in permanent physical impairment.

"Bigger is better" ads appearing on the back pages of men's magazines are totally illegitimate. Ignore them, and instead be happy with your penis. If it functions well, you have nothing to worry about. Treat it as a friend. Protect it from mutilation. The saddest men I see in my practice are those who have been subjected to phalloplasty (the surgical enhancement of the penis) for the purpose of increasing length or girth. Putting an implant into a breast is easy because it is one size and does not grow with excitement; likewise the nose can be added to, moved, or upturned because it is a static organ.

In contrast, the penis, when aroused, can grow to ten times its resting size! We have not yet discovered a way of implanting a material that will expand and contract and at the same time be physiologically and aesthetically pleasing.

There is just one safe and foolproof method for *instant* penile enlargement:

Step 1: Go to your local stationery store.

Step 2: Buy a large magnifying glass.

Step 3: Hold it over your organ, and look down through the glass. *Voila!* The Instant Penis Enlarger (IPE)!

Chapter 3

Erection and Ejaculation

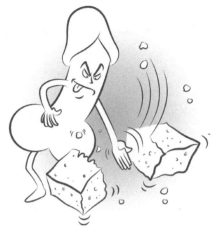

Like a two-headed Hindu god, the penis has the unique charac-teristic of fulfilling two necessary roles. It creates life by propel-ling semen toward fertile ovaries, and it preserves life by expelling toxic substances from the body in the form of urine. Both functions (which cannot take place at the same time, thanks to some efficient engineering) are carried out through the urethra.

Both functions of the penis are vital. It is interesting to note that, medically speaking, if a man were to lose his penis, he could still uri-nate, but he could no longer copulate.

Let me dispel two common misconceptions. The penis is not a mus-cle. The only muscles in the penis are the smooth muscles of the blood vessels. Despite the colloquial term for an erection—boner—there are no bones in the penis. Beneath the skin, which is extremely sensitive (especially the part we call the head or glans, so named because the an-cients thought it looked like an acorn), the penis is composed of three cylinders made up of spongy tissue.

One of these cylinders is called the corpus spongiosum. This runs along the bottom of the penis and encircles the urethra, a long canal running from the bladder all the way through the penis to the meatus, which is the hole (sometimes humorously referred to as the "eye") at the tip of the organ. It is through the urethra and out of the meatus that the penis achieves success in both of its jobs.

The other two cylinders run side by side along the upper part of the penis. They take up most of the space inside the organ. These tubular compartments, called the corpora cavernosa, consist of spongelike tissue filled with blood vessels and tiny chambers called sinusoids. If you were to look at these corpora through a microscope, you would think you were seeing an aerial view of a delta with its rivers and tributaries. Each tube is surrounded by a tough fibrous sheath (tunica). The tunica joins forces with the interior blood vessels to form an erection. The absolute interior volume, limited by the rigid tunica, or coat, dictates the size of an erect penis.

Erections: Whatever Turns You On

Erections are the result of a complex process that involves the endocrine, muscular, vascular, and neurological systems. Each of these systems is affected by psychological and emotional factors. We do not know all the intricate dynamics of *how* erections come and go. We know even less about the all-important brain-penis axis.

We do, however, understand many of the essentials. The penis gets hard in a series of distinct steps. The first reaction occurs when the nerves are stimulated, causing microscopic blood vessels in the corpora to dilate. This is *arousal*. The factors that excite any given man at any particular time are enormously varied and idiosyncratic. As the pioneering sex researcher Alfred Kinsey wrote, "There is nothing more characteristic of sexual response than the fact that it is not the same in any two individuals."[1] Whether stimulation begins with something a man sees, hears, smells, feels, or imagines, the brain determines the level of arousal. The complex neural connections between the brain and the penis are difficult to define and to quantify. The link is so intimate, immediate, and responsive, it is as if the penis has eyes, ears, and a nose. Certainly, it seems that way to an aroused man.

The penis is an exquisitely sensitive organ, particularly the glans and the shaft, and responds most dramatically to *touch*. Exactly what kind is entirely a matter of individual preference, conditioning, and circumstances. Some men like a soft, gentle touch, while others prefer a vigorous, perhaps even rough, stroke. Some men respond to the friction of a dry touch, while others favor a moist one. Some find slow, rhythmic movement a turnon, while others go wild over rapid, irregular motion. Some like all these touches to different degrees at different times.

The penis also perks up when other parts of the body are touched erotically: the thighs, the buttocks, the abdomen, the neck, the lips, and other erogenous zones. Your penis can also get aroused when you touch the right part of someone else's body. In other words, the penis has an extensive sense of touch that is necessary for arousal and also difficult to precisely define.

With the exception of men who have moral or religious objections and those with irrational phobias, I have never met a man who did not respond to oral contact. It is not just the texture of the lips and tongue on the penis, it is not just the psychological charge of having your partner perform such an intimate and generous act, but it is the actual physical effect of sucking. Sucking creates a vacuum, and a vacuum creates negative pressure within the corpora, drawing blood into the organ. That inflow of blood creates an erection.

The penis also has a sense of *smell*. As a young man, I had a particularly memorable sexual encounter with a woman who always wore a perfume with a distinct scent. To this day, whenever I catch a whiff of that perfume, I can do little to keep my pants from bursting at the seams. And the penis responds not just to man-made scents—it also responds to the perfumes of nature. Whatever seductive aromas fill the air in springtime, they surely play a role in turning a young man's fancy to love.

Many researchers believe that chemical substances known as pheromones stimulate the sexual response. Pheromones are secreted from a woman's skin and vagina. Such pheromones can stimulate a sexual response in males simply through the olfactory sense, with the invisible signals affecting women just as much as men. This natural aphrodisiac is nature's way of ensuring that male and female animals reproduce.

Also consider the impact of *sound*: romantic melodies; erotic rhythms; a gentle surf; a breeze rustling through the trees outside the bedroom window; sweet, erotic words whispered in your ear, "I want you so badly," "You're so sexy," "Do it to me." The penis responds as if it had ears of its own.

Taste also plays a part. Think of juicy tropical fruits, ice cubes, ice cream, ice *anything*, and, of course, your lover's sweat and saliva.

Visual stimulation is also vital. Whether your taste is Frederick's of Hollywood or Victoria's Secret, *Soldier of Fortune, Field & Stream, Playboy*, or *Playgirl* magazine, whether it's tight jeans or a diaphanous skirt, a skimpy bikini or a beach towel wrapped around a mystery, your penis responds to what you see or to the prospect of what you *might* see.

These are the senses, but the mind and emotions also play a crucial part in arousal. The same stimuli that work like magic on one occasion may elicit indifference on another, depending on your mood and the psychological undercurrents at that moment. The strokes, scents, and sights of a person you love, or one you have been lusting after, will produce vastly different effects than the strokes, scents, and sights of someone you cannot stand. Arousal can occur with no help from the senses at all. *Imagination* is often sufficient (and often required).

Tumescence: Stand Up and Be Counted

Whatever the source of arousal, what occurs during an erection is a complex physiological reaction involving nerves, muscles, blood vessels, and hormones. When the brain decides it is time for the penis to stand up and be counted, signals travel to the lumbar area (lower back) of the spinal cord. From there, messages are dispatched along a network of nerves to the penis. The tiny muscles within the walls of the penile arteries are ordered to relax. This opens up the corpora channels and allows more blood to flow into the flaccid penis. Blood is *always* flowing into the penis from the rest of the body, entering in relatively small amounts and then flowing back out through the veins at a more or less steady pace. Most of the time, the penis stays soft. When you are aroused, however, blood gets pumped to where it is needed, gushing into the penis at six to eight times its normal rate.

The penis then becomes engorged. The arteries distend. The small sinusoids fill up, and the corpora expand like balloons, pressing against the tunica in which they are encased. As a result, the penis not only gets bigger, it gets stiffer and more erect. The action is similar to a fire hose that turns from limp and bendable to hard and rigid as it fills with water. Just how big and how rigid the penis becomes depends on how much *potential* volume the corpora were granted by heredity. It also depends on how filled up they become. This, in turn, depends on complex mental and physical factors.

Still, it's vital to remember: *the volume of the corpora is determined by genetics and cannot be medically altered.*

In one of nature's most marvelous and elegant arrangements, the penis *stays* hard because the blood that has flooded into it causes tumescence (the swelling that creates an erection). Once the blood flows in, it does not flow out. Unless impeded by a physical abnormality or a psychological inhibition, the outflow of blood through the venous system is held in check by a valvelike mechanism. This allows the penis to remain hard long enough to accomplish its goal. It is as if the traffic lanes going into a parking lot were widened to allow more cars to enter, but once the cars were in, those lanes were blocked off, preventing traffic from flowing back out.

When ejaculation occurs, or when arousal is interrupted (the phone rings, you get nervous, or you are otherwise distracted) the result is detumescence. Detumescence is the release of blood from the corpora. During this process, the smooth muscles around the sinusoids and small arteries contract, and the roadblocks in the venous system open, allowing blood to flow back out and the penis to quickly and efficiently become flaccid.

Orgasms: Come Again?

Nature designed the mechanism of erection for procreation. The reflex of ejaculation follows erection, not to be confused with orgasm, even though the two usually, but not always, go together.

Orgasm refers to the intense feeling of pleasure and release felt at the climax of sexual excitement. Orgasm is mainly neurological in nature, an electrochemical event centered in the areas of the brain that govern pleasure. In our laboratories, we can trigger an orgasm in animals by stimulating the brain in the right way. Most of the time, men have orgasms when they ejaculate. This is referred to colloquially as coming. Most men have had the disconcerting experience of ejaculating without the pleasurable sensation of orgasm. This may have happened when, as adolescents, they were overwhelmed by excitement and anxiety and came in their pants. Conversely, some men have experienced orgasm without ejaculation. Some esoteric Eastern sex practices can accomplish this. Many of my elderly patients have also experienced it, to their considerable chagrin. This is not uncommon in the elderly age group.

Ejaculation is discharge of semen through the penis. This occurs through a reflex action involving a number of body parts.

Semen: From Whence It Comes

The sticky, milky-white ejaculate fluid is not produced exclusively in the testicles. It is the contribution of three organs: the testicles, the seminal vesicles, and the prostate.

The testicles provide the smallest amount, but the most important part, of this fluid—sperm. In a normal man, anywhere from eighty to six hundred million sperm cells accompany each ejaculation and are sent in search of a fertile egg to impregnate. Most fascinating is that those millions of sperm cells constitute only a miniscule percentage of the total volume of ejaculate.

Sperm travels from each testicle through a pair of tubes called the vas deferens. The sperm is then stored in the seminal vesicles, two pouches that stick out like pennant flags in a stiff wind behind the prostate, located near the point where the urethra emerges from the bladder.

There the sperm is mixed with the rest of the seminal fluid, which is a medium to transport the sperm. Some of the fluid is manufactured in the seminal vesicles, and the remaining portion comes from the prostate gland, an oval-shaped organ about the size of a plum located at the neck of the bladder and surrounding the urethra. Only men have prostates. The prostate not only contributes to the content of the semen but also facilitates the process of ejaculation itself. It helps shut off the flow of urine from the bladder so that semen alone enters the penis.

The complex products of the testicles, prostate, and seminal vesicles form the final composition of the fluid that is ejaculated at the climax of the sex act.

Another secretion is actually the first to emerge—a clear, sticky fluid manufactured in the bulbourethral glands. These glands are called Cowper's glands (named after the seventeenth-century English surgeon William Cowper). The Cowper's glands are about the size of peas and are located just under the prostate. Small drops of the Cowper's fluid typically appear at the tip of the penis during the arousal stage. Some men confuse this with ejaculate, causing them to believe that they are ejaculating too quickly and to panic. Although it is not ejaculate, do not make the mistake of assuming that the fluid contains no sperm cells; it may contain some, and only one sperm cell is needed to fertilize an egg. The purpose of the fluid from the Cowper's gland is to help lubricate the vagina.

As you can see, this masterfully designed system does not miss a trick.

The Point of No Return

With sufficient stimulation to an erect penis, the reflex action of ejaculation is eventually triggered. The amount of time it takes depends on the individual and on the circumstances. The sensation of pleasure involved also may vary. A man might experience fireworks and ejaculate very quickly, or he might require an extended period of stimulation in order to achieve climax. The differences in the intensity and pleasure of orgasm are mediated in the brain, entailing psychological and emotional factors. What takes place *physically* during ejaculation is always the same. This is true with minor variations—whether a man is masturbating in a closet or making love under a tropical waterfall with the partner of his dreams.

When a certain level of excitement is reached, a complex chain of nerve impulses signals the muscles in the pelvic floor to contract. These muscles are located in the perineum, the area between the back of the scrotum and the bottom of the rectum (often referred to as the taint, as in "'tain't in the front and 'tain't in the back"). These contractions close the neck of the bladder and open the ejaculatory ducts. Sperm and seminal fluid can then enter the urethra, where the components are combined. These pelvic contractions are accompanied by muscle contractions in other parts of the body (such as the lower back and abdomen) and by an increase in the heart and respiratory rates, making ejaculation a whole-body phenomenon.

At this point, when the contractions of the perineal muscles forcefully start to move the semen on its route through the penis, men feel the sensations that tell them they are about to ejaculate. From this point on, ejaculation is inevitable. It is a pure reflex that cannot be stopped. The ejaculate is powerfully propelled from the back of the urethra through the penis and out the tip. It squirts out in several jellylike clumps, which quickly liquefy into an opaque fluid, allowing the sperm to swim to the ovaries. Exactly how much is ejaculated varies. The older you get, the less semen is produced. Ejaculation is also influenced by the length of time since the previous ejaculation. Statistically, the amount of seminal fluid per ejaculate ranges from two to five cubic centimeters and averages three cubic centimeters, which is about a teaspoon. The volume decreases with age because the body simply produces less. The forcefulness of ejaculation also decreases with age due to a natural decline in muscular strength and changes in the vascular system. Still, no matter the amount or forcefulness, the mechanism is exactly the same, and no real correlation exists between the volume of ejaculate and the amount of pleasure that is experienced.

Some men complain to me that their sex lives are lousy because they do not ejaculate as much as they used to. When I tell them that *everyone* produces less semen as they age and that it has nothing to do with a person's level of sexual pleasure, they either start enjoying sex again because they are relieved of this self-imposed psychological burden, or they are forced to focus on the *real* problem, which can be anything from a conflict with a partner to a correctable medical condition.

A relationship does exist between the strength and duration of the perineal contractions and the intensity of pleasure. Chapter 15 offers exercises to strengthen the perineal muscles, but remember, any difference in the satisfaction from one ejaculation to another is centered overwhelmingly between your ears, not between your legs or in your perineum.

A particular orgasm might *feel* especially satisfying because of the intensity of the emotions involved or the partner's sexual skills or other circumstances surrounding the experience. If an orgasm that is accompanied by a large amount of semen *does* feel unusually intense, the reason is most likely that the man has gone a long time between ejaculations. The more extended this time gap is, the more fluid builds up in the seminal vesicles. The overdistention of these storage pouches creates the heightened sexual tension that is released in an explosive orgasm.

The Refractory Period: I Want to Be Alone

As soon as ejaculation is completed, heartbeat, blood pressure, and respiratory rate gradually slow to resting levels. You feel sated and relaxed, and perhaps sleepy. The scrotum, which reflexively contracts during sexual arousal, and the testes, which rise up within the scrotal sac, relax into their usual positions. The penis, as the blood drains out, reverts to its flaccid state. It is as if having worked so hard, the penis wants to retreat into solitude. The head of the penis becomes extremely sensitive and does not want to be touched or sucked. It might even burn or hurt if it makes contact with anything. After ejaculation, the penis in effect dons a neon sign that reads, "Leave me alone!" This is a refractory period, a time when the male body restores its energy before it can once again become aroused and when no amount of stimulation will produce an erection or ejaculation.

Exactly how long it takes for sexual function to be restored varies considerably from one man to another. Any man will notice distinct variations in his refractory period depending on his partner, the circumstances of the sexual encounter, and such physical factors as fatigue and general health. The two main variables that determine the length of the refractory period are age and the length of time since the previous ejaculation. Generally speaking, the older the man, the longer the refractory period. The same man who at nineteen was ready to go five minutes after ejaculating might need an hour at age forty or a full day at age sixty. Conversely, a man who has gone without sex for a long period of time will be restored much more quickly than if he has just ejaculated for the tenth time in two days.

The refractory period is nature's way of making sure men do not waste their energy when they have no semen to contribute. During this rest phase the seminal vesicles are refilled. These vesicles act like a reservoir with a feedback system. When they are empty, or the volume of seminal fluid is low, the body starts producing more. As the supply of semen is replenished, the seminal vesicles become distended. When they are filled up with fluid again, seminal production is curtailed, and the refractory period is over.

The distended seminal vesicles trigger a neurological signal that produces a sense of pressure in the perineum. That produces the common feeling of being "frisky." Now that the refractory period is over, and the gates are open, the penis perks up, raises its head, and once again starts calling attention to itself.

This is the basic anatomy of erection and ejaculation.

Chapter 4

Medical Conditions That Affect Penis Power

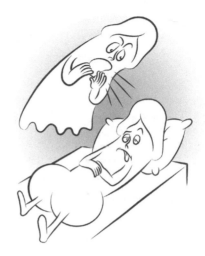

A lmost all the sexual problems men report to me fall into three basic categories: problems with desire, difficulties with erection, and complications with ejaculation.

Concerns about diminished desire usually come from middle-aged or elderly men who are distressed that they do not crave sex as much as they once did. Concerns about ejaculation present in two ways: too fast (premature ejaculation) or too slow (retarded ejaculation). I hear "quick-on-the-trigger" or premature ejaculation complaints mainly from younger men. The too-slow or retarded ejaculation variety comes from their elders. Problems with desire are rarely treatable medical disorders, except in cases with low testosterone levels, certain psychological or emotionally caused ejaculation troubles, and other rare exceptions.

In most instances, these issues are treated by psychological and behavioral therapy. In many cases, those patients who have such complaints do not actually have a problem. They are simply misinformed about what is to be reasonably expected from their bodies.

In Freud's heyday, impotence was assumed to be a purely psycho-logical problem. Most men who could not obtain satisfactory erections were psychoanalyzed to find the deep, dark roots of their neurosis. Then the medical world learned that erection problems could also be caused by physical disorders.

This significant discovery led doctors to develop sophisticated tools used to distinguish between organic impotence and psychogenic penis weakness. These instruments are particularly useful in identifying erectile dysfunction caused by nonorganic psychological and situational factors. In cases where the cause is a true medical or biological condition, modern medical technology allows us to make a precise diagnosis and formulate a focused treatment plan.

The reasons that an erection does not occur as desired, or last as long as expected, are even more complex and varied than the reasons it works properly. This chapter focuses on the medical conditions that affect penis power, beginning with a few general points worth considering regarding both the organic and inorganic causes of penis weakness.

Impotence: "My Friend Has This Problem . . ."

No greater symbol of masculinity exists than an erection, an anatomical equivalent of wealth, power, and strength—the "rescuing the damsel in distress," "winning the ball game," "defeating the bad guy in time to save the village," all wrapped into one shaft of flesh and blood. Nothing carries with it more humiliation or self-recrimination than the failure to achieve an erection, a condition known as erectile dysfunction.

Few things are more difficult for a man to admit than that he is having an erection problem. Most men put off telling even their physicians for as long as they can, sometimes until it is too late to easily correct the situation. Most women have great difficulty in understanding the depths of humiliation a man feels when, in the midst of passionate foreplay, his penis does not get erect. Women also have difficulty understanding the even more humiliating situation when an erect penis suddenly and without warning goes limp.

When a woman's genitalia do not lubricate, she can reach for the K-Y Jelly or her partner can use saliva. Even if she is not terribly aroused, a woman can proceed with intercourse. If she wants to, she can always *pretend* to be passionate. A man without an erection has no such fall-back position. With his penis drooping like a flag on a windless day, no artifice can compensate. This is a nightmare worse than dropping a touchdown pass in the end zone or striking out with the bases loaded. Even if it happens just once, the event can be devastating. Few men are able to shrug it off. When it happens more than once, the shake-up to self-esteem is high. Most men fail to realize that they *should* shrug it off, that this happens from time to time to every man.

When a male patient comes into my office and reluctantly admits that he is having problems, I first try to make him feel comfortable and safe so that we can speak openly and honestly about his situation. Usually, the conversation starts with some equivalent of the phrase: "Doc, my friend has this problem." Now, we both know who this "friend" really is.

I quickly try to let him know that I understand it is *his* predicament, and that no matter the details, we will straighten everything out. Once I establish rapport and trust, I take a medical history. The first detail I want to know is whether my patient's problem with erections is of recent origin or if it has been going on for a long time. I then ask if the onset of the problem was sudden or if it was gradual. I ask a series of questions about his personal life, general lifestyle, and emotional state. I follow an algorithm (a preset course of medical questions) in which the patient's answers guide each subsequent question. This leads to an accurate diagnosis. You would be surprised how many men come to me in a complete penis panic only to find out that their problem is not medical, but circumstantial—a marriage in jeopardy, a business predicament, or just plain mental and physical fatigue.

If my analysis to this point has not revealed any obvious *situational* cause, my line of inquiry turns to medical factors. When the penis fails to perform properly and when psychological factors are ruled out, the diagnosis falls into the clinical category of organic impotence. Even though only a small number of the men who come to me are in this category, my first responsibility is to search for a possible medical cause of the problem. Before embarking on a sophisticated *medical* evaluation, I have to be convinced that the patient is, in fact, physically incapable of having an erection. This is often accomplished with one question.

Take the case of a fifty-year-old executive who came to me with a minor irritation on his scrotal skin (the skin covering the testicles). I prescribed a topical ointment. I then listened as this aggressive, no-nonsense mover and shaker gazed at the floor and sheepishly told me the real reason for his visit to my office: "Doc, I just cannot get it up lately." He felt fine otherwise and was not under any exceptional degree of stress.

At that moment, my secretary buzzed to tell me that the lab assistant had stopped by to pick up a blood sample. Knowing that this assistant was a beautiful young woman, I seized the opportunity to use a visual aid to solve this diagnostic problem.

When the assistant entered the exam area, I handed her the sample, and as she swayed out the door, I watched my patient eye her shapely figure.

"If she came on to you, do you think you would have any problem rising to the occasion?" I asked.

"Are you kidding, Doc?" said the patient. "When do we start?"

The patient's "medical" problem was solved because it never existed! His penis weakness was the result of problems within his marital bedroom, not the result of an anatomic malfunction of his organ. A remark like his does not constitute scientific proof, but in this patient's case, other evidence was in place. He confessed to having had a recent dalliance with a woman he met on a business trip. During the affair, he performed adequately. From that fact alone, I determined he was not physically impaired. I suggested that he and his wife might want to see a marriage counselor.

For most patients, the question of whether a penis problem is physical or mental cannot be settled in an interview. I have to use reliable, *objective* criteria. I have a method that is foolproof.

Fact: all *healthy* males get erections during their sleep. This happens every night without exception. Each episode lasts about half an hour, although the penis is not fully erect the entire time. All healthy men, regardless of age, get these nocturnal erections three to five times a night.

They occur in cycles, separated by one to two hours. Most coincide with the REM (rapid eye movement) stage of sleep, the period during which dreaming occurs. But these erections are totally nonsexual in nature; even infants have them.

I do not want to create the false impression that a twenty-year-old sleeping penis acts the same as its sixty-year-old counterpart. The total duration of nocturnal erections is age related, longest during the teenage years, after which they gradually decline. Normal, healthy men in their eighties still have three or four erections per night. On the average, the penis of a medically fit man is erect more than one hundred minutes a night! Urologists do not know the purpose of these nocturnal erections or what their function is in the sleep process. Thankfully, however, they give doctors an important diagnostic tool.

If a man has normal erections during sleep, we assume he is anatomically and physiologically capable of having good erections during sex. We can then safely conclude that his penis weakness is not rooted in any organic condition; rather, it is psychological in origin. Conversely, if the patient does *not* have normal sleep erections, we conclude that some organic condition is impeding the process, and the diagnosis is organic impotence.

If one of my patients happens to wake up in the middle of the night and finds his penis erect, or if he has an erection when he wakes up in the morning (the condition often referred to as morning wood or a piss hard-on because it is often accompanied by the need to urinate), he has the luxury of knowing that his penis is in good working order. Urologists, however, have a more convincing way to make this determination: a diagnostic procedure called the nocturnal penile tumescence (NPT) test.

To perform this test we give the patient a simple take-home kit consisting of a state-of-the-art gadget with loops that look like a small pair of blood pressure cuffs. One loop is placed around the penis at the base and one just under the glans. Comfortable enough to sleep with, but secure enough not to fall off, the gauges are attached by wire to a meter hooked up to a polygraph printer, just like those used in lie detector tests.

If the patient's penis enlarges as it would with a normal nocturnal erection, the pressure inside the cuffs increases. This change registers in graph form on the recording device. We can actually measure the increase in diameter and the degree of rigidity of the penis. We can also measure the frequency and duration of the erections. This simple device tells me whether a patient is *physically* capable of achieving a satisfactory erection. Regardless of the outcome of the test, my patients invariably feel better after using the kit because now, at last, the mystery and torment have been solved.

These patients are either relieved to discover that they can, in fact, have an erection and nothing is medically wrong, or they are relieved to find out that the problem is physical and not mental. Once I know the problem is physical, I can proceed to evaluate the actual nature of the disorder and outline an appropriate treatment plan. Before we had sophisticated monitoring devices, I relied on a simple, homemade procedure that patients who are intimidated by machines can still use. Take a roll of postage stamps, and wrap it around your penis before you go to sleep (keeping in mind the escalating cost of postage). If when you awaken in the morning the perforation between the stamps is torn, there is a good chance you had an erection during the night. The postage stamp test, though scientifically crude, is fairly reliable.

If the patient fails to get an adequate nighttime erection, proceeding with a complete urologic evaluation is the next step. Thanks to some remarkable medical advances, men who suffer from physical disorders can be treated. In the old days, such men might have spent years in psychotherapy while their self-esteem and penis power plummeted to even greater depths. The key to a successful treatment plan is to obtain an accurate diagnosis, and in most cases, urologists can determine the cause right in their offices. Organic disorders fall into three basic categories: neurological, vascular, and hormonal. Organic causes are responsible for a relatively small percentage of erectile dysfunction cases that I encounter.

The Nerve of It: Neurological Disorders

Some patients are incapable of generating or sustaining an erection because of impairments in the complex network of nerves that make an erection possible. In almost all such cases, the impotence is a symptom of a preexisting neurological disorder such as multiple sclerosis, Parkinson's disease, cervical disc disease, or spinal cord tumors or injuries. In addition, chronic conditions such as long-term alcoholism and advanced diabetes can lead to damage of the peripheral nerves and can impair erections.

When nocturnal erections do not occur and a patient's medical history reveals any of these disorders, a neurological failure is suspected. To verify this, I sometimes perform a simple exam called the bulbocavernosus reflex test. I insert a gloved finger into the patient's anal sphincter. With my other hand, I gently squeeze the tip of the penis. If the reflex arc is working properly, the anal sphincter will contract firmly against my examining finger. With this simple test, I can determine whether or not the reflex arc, which is necessary for erection, is functional.

Fortunately, some of the neurological conditions that cause penis weakness are correctable. If a damaged cervical disc is surgically corrected or a spinal tumor is removed, a patient has a good chance of recovering normal erectile function. Sadly, though, most neurological causes of penis failure are not permanently correctable and are outside the urologist's expertise. With new developments in the field of erectile dysfunction such as injection therapy, the use of penile prosthetic devices, and especially the safe use of oral erectile dysfunction drugs, these organic conditions are often successfully treatable.

When It Cannot Go with the Flow: Vascular Disorders

Of all the *medical* causes of erectile dysfunction, by far the most common are vascular diseases. A lot of problems can be caused by an obstruction in the arteries that bring blood to the penis or by leaks in the venous system that result when the blood in the shaft drains out prematurely. In other words, if not enough blood enters your penis or not enough blood is held there, your penis cannot stay erect.

I always look in my patient's medical history for evidence of cardio-vascular disease: high blood pressure, chest pain (angina), or pain in the legs after walking or exercising (claudication), all symptoms related to conditions that block the blood vessels of the body and, consequently, those that serve the penis.

Through a calculated discussion with a patient, I can get a good idea of whether or not to look further for possible vascular disturbances. In the past, tests identifying vascular defects in the erection process were time consuming and difficult to perform. They were even more difficult to interpret. That has changed. We now have several simple and highly accurate techniques for identifying vascular problems.

An especially sophisticated method for identifying arterial insuffi-ciency is the Doppler pulse-wave analysis. This instrument produces an ultrasound beam that we direct toward the blood vessels in the penis. The motion of the blood cells bounces a signal back to the instrument, and the signal responds to the volume of blood flowing through the vessel. The signal is either amplified into an audible sound or recorded as waves onto a chart. The procedure is noninvasive, painless, and ex-tremely precise. Without having to attach gadgets to the penis itself, we can measure the blood flow through individual arteries.

Still more advanced, but more invasive, is a method called penile arteriography. In this process, we inject a dye into the artery that sup-plies blood to the penis and then monitor the blood flow with x-ray equipment that is sensitive to the dye. This is by far the most accu-rate way to assess the minute arteries that supply blood to the penis during erection. We do not perform this procedure routinely, since it requires anesthetizing the patient and injecting the dye directly into a very small artery, sometimes producing unwanted complications. I re-serve this procedure for a few select cases, such as patients with major pelvic injuries or isolated arterial damage that might be amenable to surgical repair.

A Little Prick for a Big Reward: Injectable Drugs

In the early 1980s, a revolutionary technique was introduced with major implications for both the diagnosis and treatment of erectile dysfunction. This technique entails injecting specific vasoactive drugs (drugs that dilate the penile arteries) into the penis. The drugs dramatically increase blood flow to the penis, usually producing an immediate erection regardless of mental factors. Erection will occur even in the face of significant systemic blood vessel disease.

The most commonly used injectable drugs are papaverine and prostaglandin-E1 (also known as PGE-1 or alprostadil). In my experience, the injections are the best way to screen for circulatory problems. With one simple injection, we can determine whether the arterial system is intact. The penis either gets hard or it does not. If the injection works, we then carefully instruct the patient in self-administration analogous to a diabetic injecting insulin.

If a patient gets only a partial erection or loses an erection when he changes position, I might also suspect problems with blood flow *out* of the penis—a venous leak. In some cases, blood flows into the penis normally but is not held in the corpora within the shaft long enough to sustain erection. This usually occurs because the valve mechanism in the veins is not working adequately to trap the blood. New ultrasound technology enables us to diagnose a venous leak easily and effectively.

These harmless and painless methods for measuring the dynamics of penile dysfunction represent medical miracles. Now that we can measure the blood flow through each and every vessel in the penis, we can accurately diagnose blood vessel obstructions and leaks. Even more amazing is that we can take precise steps to correct these problems. In chapter 6 I describe in detail the use of papaverine and prostaglandin-E1 injections to restore declining penis power, especially in aging men.

When Something Is Not Quite Right: Hormonal Disorders

The most common endocrine disease associated with penis failure is diabetes, a syndrome characterized by the abnormal secretion of insulin. Insulin precisely regulates the amount of circulating blood sugar. Diabetes is a major cause of generalized arteriosclerosis (hardening of the arteries) and widespread neuropathy, a disorder that destroys nerves throughout the body, and can also cause severe damage to the blood vessels, as well as the nerves going to the penis.

A significant number of my young, diabetic, male patients experience a gradual decrease in the *sensitivity* of their penises, as well as a decline in the firmness of their erections. Tragically, many diabetics ultimately become entirely incapable of normal sexual functioning, but if the disease is diagnosed early and is properly managed with diet, oral medication, insulin injections, and regular exercise, diabetic men have a good chance of restoring strong penis power—or never having it weaken at all.

Other hormonal conditions can also affect penis power. Abnormal thyroid function, in the form of either an underactive or an overactive thyroid gland, can affect male sexual health. Another potential hormonal problem is the overproduction of the hormone prolactin. This hormone is usually a side effect of certain medications or tumors in the pituitary gland. A deficiency of the male sex hormone testosterone is another hormonal problem. In a moderate number of my patients, a simple blood-screening test might reveal abnormally low levels of testosterone. This usually makes itself known by a loss or diminution of sexual drive and desire (libido). In urologic parlance, testosterone is known as the desire drug. Most patients who develop low levels of testosterone have suffered a testicular injury or have had the mumps virus as children. Mumps can lead to orchitis, an inflammation that causes the testicles to atrophy or deteriorate, rendering them deficient in testosterone production.

This condition is also quite common in some of my older male patients. Patients who suffer from atrophy can be treated with either periodic injections of testosterone or the application of a testosterone gel or patch to the skin for transdermal absorption. Both of these methods can bring circulating testosterone up to normal levels in the body and can effectively restore the patient's full penis power. The key to diagnosing and treating these patients is to recognize testicular failure (hypogonadism) as the cause. Hypogonadism and the process of andropause (the male equivalent of menopause) are further discussed in later chapters.

Steroids: Big Biceps and Tiny Testes

I must emphasize that *there is no legitimate reason to use testosterone if the circulating blood level is already within the normal range*. Contrary to the belief of many of my patients, using testosterone will *not* improve the penis performance of someone whose testosterone level is normal to begin with. More importantly, testosterone and its derivatives, the anabolic steroids, can cause serious side effects. Through a complex feedback mechanism, the body is fine tuned to maintain just the right amount of circulating testosterone. It can use only so much of it. If a man whose testosterone level is within the normal range consumes additional amounts, either orally or by injection, a signal is sent from the pituitary gland in the brain to the testicles to produce *less* of the male hormone. If you add some from the outside, the body's computer says, "Hey, I'm getting all this extra testosterone—I'd better tell the testicles to stop producing the stuff." The result is testicular atrophy, or "tiny testes."

In my practice, I have seen several terrific male specimens—athletes and movie stars with bodies like sculpted marble. They discovered to their horror that steroids were destroying their fertility and their sex lives. Their testicles had shrunk to the size of peas. The results are simply not worth it, even for men whose fortunes depend on their muscular images. For a normal man who is not testosterone deficient, taking anabolic steroids (testosterone or its derivatives) in the hope of turning into a stud is madness.

Do Not Be Sicker Than You Really Are

The general weakness and fatigue that accompanies any illness will naturally affect your sex drive. Also, depending on the nature of the affliction and its severity, a patient's range of movement might be limited to the point where he is not able to engage in sex. In many cases, illness brings depression or despair, a feeling of inadequacy, and an image of one's body as impaired. All this can diminish penis power.

Unfortunately, many sick men give up on themselves as sexual beings because they are convinced they are no longer capable of virile, sexual activities. They might also become unreasonably fearful and refrain from all sex-related exercise that could potentially benefit their conditions. Men with arthritis, for example, sometimes abstain from sex because the pain in their joints prevents them from moving around as vigorously as they would like. They are not only depriving themselves of some much-needed and well-deserved joy, but they are also overlooking the significant ways in which sex can improve range of motion and relieve pain. My rheumatology colleagues tell me evidence has shown that people with arthritis can experience relief from pain for up to four to six hours after an orgasm.

Unfortunately, some physicians advise these patients to limit their sexual activity, or even give it up entirely, when illness strikes. A doctor who goes by the book might even tell a patient that he will never have "normal sex relations" again. What terrible advice! Patients not only get depressed when they hear this but also take it to mean that they have to retire their penises. The doctor's negative prognosis is often flawed. Not long ago, physicians told heart patients and people with back pain to avoid exercise. Today, we prescribe exercise programs for their rehabilitation and advise against being sedentary. In many cases, the same is true of sex. I advise and encourage my patients to use their penises to bring cheer to the sickbed, rather than allowing the penis to shrivel up before its time.

If your doctor tells you to abstain from exercising your penis power, get a second opinion! He or she may be misinformed or simply old fashioned. Illness might *limit* your sexuality, but it does not have to *eliminate* it. For most individuals, the solution involves learning new habits. Your condition might mean that you take longer to achieve an erection, in which case you can learn to be more patient, and your partner can learn new ways to stimulate you. If your illness makes it impossible to make love in the positions to which you are accustomed, practice new positions that do work. You might have to have sex less often or less vigorously, but you can learn to fully savor the slow and gentle sensuality that you used to hurry through.

If you have intercourse less often, you might be able to enjoy oral sex or mutual masturbation *more* often. Such changes should be viewed as opportunities for new experiences, rather than reasons to give up one of life's greatest pleasures.

Prescription Medications: Is the Pharmacist Really Your Enemy?

A television producer that I had treated for a urinary infection returned, and I could tell from his facial expression that he had not come to see me only about the infection. Whatever was on his mind wasn't something he found easy to talk about. When he finally said, "Doctor, I cannot get hard anymore," I was shocked. He had a reputation as a Casanova who took pride in his penis power. We talked for a while about his life. I explored the possibility that he, as a single man who liked a variety of partners, might feel frightened by the AIDS epidemic. No, he said, he was careful to thoroughly screen partners and always practice safe sex. I thought he might be under some stress from his profession. He assured me that wasn't the case. In fact, he loved sex as an outlet for his built-up tension.

When I took his medical history in preparation for a complete examination, I stumbled upon the answer. Since I had last seen him, he had been diagnosed with high blood pressure. The good news was that the hypertension itself was not affecting his penis power. The bad news was that the prescription medication he was taking to control it *was* having an effect on his penis power.

A number of therapeutic drugs can cause erection or ejaculation problems, even in men with excellent penis attitudes. Unfortunately, few rigorous scientific studies have been performed on the subject, so most of what we know about penis weakness associated with the use of common medicines is anecdotal or reported by manufacturers as possible side effects.

When I suspect that a drug might be responsible for a patient's problem, I do an informal test consisting of reducing the dosage or eliminating the drug entirely to see if the patient's penis power is restored. I do this with the cooperation of the primary physician and with all possible safeguards observed. In the case of the television producer, we safely lowered the dosage of his antihypertensive medicine, and he was quickly back to his old tricks.

Blood pressure medications are not the only culprits, although they are probably the most common. Sexual dysfunction is listed as a potential side effect of virtually every antihypertensive agent. These medications work in different ways to lower blood pressure, so their effects on the penis also vary. If you are taking medication for high blood pressure and suspect that it may be adversely affecting your penis power, consult your physician. You might be able to switch to a class of drugs whose ingredients will not keep you from being a superpotent man.

Other drugs that can diminish penis power include diuretics and some medications used to treat anxiety, depression, and other psychiatric disturbances. These can cause diminished libido, retarded ejaculation, or erection problems. Various ulcer medications can also cause impotency in some patients because they disrupt the production of testosterone.

Do not, however, arbitrarily give up or alter any prescription medications you are taking. If you suspect that a prescription drug is negatively affecting your penis power, consult with your physician. Reducing a dosage or stopping the use of a particular medication can cause a complicated and potentially life-threatening situation. Even a well-trained physician is not always able to tell with certainty whether a specific medication is causing the problem. Many forces, not just the medication, might be contributing to your inability to get an erection. Most patients who take hypertension medications are of advanced age, may suffer from more than one illness, may take a variety of medications, and may have other habits adversely affecting their penis power. High blood pressure alone can weaken penis power. Approximately 10 percent of patients who require antihypertensive drugs have significant penis weakness *before* starting treatment. Similarly, depression triggered by the illness itself can also cause sexual dysfunction.

The sexual side effects of the drugs have to be weighed against the consequences of the diseases themselves. In some cases, switching medications or adjusting the dosage is an easy solution. When that is not possible, living with diminished penis power might be wiser than risking aggravating a serious medical condition by disrupting its treatment.

Such decisions require delicate clinical judgment, which is why you should have a frank and thorough discussion with your physician and commit to a rigorous scrutiny of all possible options.

It's Not All Fun and Games: Recreational Drugs

Scenarios such as the one with the television producer occur not only with prescription drugs, but also with so-called recreational substances.

Drug and alcohol abuse and addiction can cause everything from temporary penis failure to long-term impotence. Some substances create the *illusion* of enhanced sexuality because they seem to take the edge off, calm you down, lower inhibitions, and produce a heightened sensitivity.

"Candy is dandy, but liquor is quicker" is a common expression. We all know the routine. You have a few drinks, and everything from your tongue to your toes loosens up. Wallflowers dance, the tongue-tied become talkative, and the sexually repressed become Lotharios. Suddenly anything and everything become possible. For those reasons, alcohol has become as much a part of lovemaking for some people as soft lights. Moderate, judicious drinking is not dangerous. If moderate consumption reduces anxiety, slows you down, and delays ejaculation a bit, alcohol can be a boon to penis power. Unfortunately, if you overdo it, your penis will poop out when it ought to pop out. Abusing alcohol or illicit substances makes becoming aroused more difficult—delaying ejaculation, reducing the pleasure and intensity of orgasms, and greatly diminishing penis rigidity.

In my practice, nearly 50 percent of the chronic alcoholics I have counseled experience either total or partial impotence. The short-term effects appear to be based on alcohol's sedative action on the central nervous system. The long-term or chronic effects include severe nerve damage of the kind that can diminish penis sensitivity and permanently impair the ability to get an erection.

Many patients have told me that marijuana enhances their penis power. Some studies have indicated that marijuana can, in fact, slow the ejaculatory process.[1] For a younger man who might be quick on the trigger, this can be perceived as "enhanced" potency because marijuana might lower inhibitory mechanisms, reduce anxiety, and heighten erotic sensations. However, I recommend extreme caution about jumping to the conclusion that marijuana is an aphrodisiac. Since it is a mind-altering substance, its effect on sexuality is most likely illusory. Research shows that marijuana's negative effects are similar to those of alcohol. I suspect that, like alcohol, in the long run marijuana use would be hostile to penis power. There is good evidence that long-term marijuana smoking weakens overall fitness and reduces energy and motivation.[2]

In addition to alcohol and marijuana, cocaine can be detrimental to penis power. When Cole Porter wrote that he doesn't get a kick from cocaine, he might not have been thinking about sex, but where penis power is concerned, cocaine is certainly no kick. In the short term, cocaine has an excitatory effect on the nervous system and can stimulate arousal and make every sensory experience *seem* more intense. In the long run, cocaine will turn a superpotent man into a super-*wimp*. Pharmacologically, it decreases the reuptake of the neurotransmitter catecholamine, a chemical that is essential for the adequate completion of the erection process. Failure to get and maintain erections is a common complaint from cocaine abusers. No man who aspires to penis power should go anywhere near this drug.

As for other illicit drugs, no superpotent man should ever use them. Amphetamines certainly kill libido, ejaculatory function, and erections, and the long-term sexual impact is devastating. This is also true for narcotics such as heroin, codeine, and Demerol and painkillers such as Vicodin, Valium, and Oxycontin. Users experience a drastic reduction in libido, as well as chronic difficulty with erections.

One more drug has long been associated with mating rituals—nicotine. As if there were not enough reasons to stop smoking (or never start), consider this: smoking has been linked to penis weakness. Several studies have demonstrated that ED is more prevalent among smokers than among nonsmokers. In one study, animals exposed to tobacco smoke or intravenous nicotine were unable to produce or maintain erections.[3] The simple scientific reason for this is that nicotine constricts blood vessels. When you smoke, the supply of arterial blood to the penis is reduced, making it more difficult to get a firm erection.

If you want to be a man of penis power, just say no to drugs and nicotine.

Premature Ejaculation

Premature ejaculation (PE) is one of the most common forms of sexual dysfunction in men today. The true cause and frequency remain unknown, but PE affects more than 30 percent of the male population and is consistent across all age groups. It is, however, more common in my younger patients. Unlike erectile dysfunction, which increases with age, PE is generally not affected by age, marital status, race, or ethnicity. Some men face this problem from adolescence through adulthood. It has historically been perceived as a sexual dysfunction of psychological versus organic origin. Only within the past decade or so have organic etiologies of PE been explored.

PE is a nuisance that many men do not realize they can fix. Sexual therapists and urologists recommend a number of self-help techniques that have proven to be very effective. Recently, there has also been significant research into the development of off-label pharmacological therapies that can help delay ejaculation.

Unfortunately, no oral or topical medication is currently approved by the Food and Drug Administration (FDA) for premature ejaculation. However, a number of therapies are still being tested that are widely available over the counter. The most common of these is Promescent, a lidocaine spray that is used prior to intercourse. One product available by prescription but off label is EMLA cream, a combination of lidocaine and prilocaine, which is applied to the penis about forty minutes before intercourse. EMLA should be washed off before intercourse; otherwise, it desensitizes a woman's clitoris and vagina.

According to the American Urological Association, urologists use as many as five definitions for PE to assess a patient. A substantial amount of agreement exists among the various definitions. These state that premature ejaculation is the inability to control ejaculation sufficiently for both partners to enjoy sexual interaction and is usually marked by a persistent or recurrent onset of orgasm and ejaculation with minimal stimulation before, on, or shortly after penetration. It occurs before the person wishes to ejaculate. This is usually compounded by distress and frustration within a sexual relationship.

PE is not life-threatening, but it does affect quality of life. In a recent survey of men with and without PE, 90 percent of those surveyed ranked fulfilling a partner's sexual needs as very or extremely important.[4]

Men who have a problem with PE find it increasingly difficult to satisfy their partners through intercourse. Their partners feel increasingly frustrated, and this creates a negative chain reaction. Coupled with poor communication and a lack of awareness, PE can cause severe rifts in an otherwise healthy, intimate relationship.

If You Need Help, Come and Get It

Surprisingly, only about 25 percent of men with PE receive treatment.[5] I find the most common barriers to seeking treatment are embarrassment and reluctance to admit the problem exists. The public has the misperception that PE is *transient* and solely psychological. Add to that the lack of knowledge regarding the availability of pharmacological therapies and the common confusion regarding the difference between erectile dysfunction (ED) and premature ejaculation (PE), and it is no wonder that PE remains, for the most part, a hidden problem. To fully understand what is happening in men who experience PE, we must look at the normal physiology of male sexual response. As discussed, achieving a normal erection is a complex event involving vascular and neurological phenomena with hormonal and psychological influences. Abnormalities in any of these areas can lead to ED or PE.

Ejaculation and erection usually occur together, even though they are not regulated by the same mechanisms, and one can occur without the other. During each sexual act, ejaculation is initially under some control until one reaches that level of excitation we call the point of ejaculatory inevitability, when ejaculation becomes completely reflexive and out of one's control.

Interestingly, the sensation that occurs with orgasm is not reflexive. Orgasm is a distinct cognitive and emotional event. The normal male sexual response follows a cycle with four phases: excitement (desire), plateau (arousal), ejaculation and orgasm, and a refractory period during which a man cannot ejaculate again. Although the cause of PE remains largely unknown, it is believed that the sexual response cycle in men with PE involves a disruption of the normal curve of ejaculatory response, usually characterized by a steep excitement phase with a shortened plateau phase leading to premature ejaculation and a rapid refractory phase.

Anxiety also appears to play an important role since it activates the sympathetic nervous system and lowers the ejaculatory threshold. I see problematic PE in my patients who are sexually inexperienced or in those who have infrequent sex, problematic relationships, or a poor understanding of the sexual response cycle.

To put this whole picture into numbers, the average length of intercourse for men with PE is under two minutes. For men with normal ejaculatory response, it is somewhere between seven and a half and nine minutes. Don't we all wish it were longer? If you are concerned that you may be suffering from PE, ask yourself the following questions:

- Are you dissatisfied with your sex life because of your lack of staying power?
- During the majority of times you have sex, do you ejaculate before you wish?

If you answered yes or if you identify with the time comparison, and PE is a problem for you, solutions are available. Urologists, unlike most others in the healthcare community, have the expertise to make available a wide variety of topical and oral off-label agents that can be used to prolong your staying power.

Off the Record

Some of my patients try self-help approaches for PE, including pre-coital masturbation and the utilization of multiple condoms. Self-help approaches also include engaging in distraction techniques (mental exercises) during foreplay and intercourse and aggressive thrusting during intercourse to speed their partner's satisfaction. Many of these techniques can actually exacerbate PE, helping the patient deliberately ignore the sexual sensations needed to establish ejaculatory control.

Currently, pharmacological strategies used off label for the treatment of PE include topical local anesthetics, PDE-5 inhibitors (oral erectile dysfunction drugs such as Viagra), and the chronic (daily or regular) use of a class of drugs designed to treat depression called selective serotonin reuptake inhibitors (SSRIs). These drugs can be taken either daily or on demand, and the goals are similar to the self-help treatments—the objective is to extend the plateau period and delay ejaculation, affording greater control over ejaculation and ultimately leading to greater sexual satisfaction for both the patient and his partner.

SSRIs were initially formulated for continuous daily use to treat depression. Surprisingly, many patients noted the retardation or delay of ejaculation while taking them. Of the SSRIs, the most commonly used are Paxil, Prozac, and Zoloft. Each is effective in delaying ejaculation, but Paxil has been found to exert the greatest effect. The optimal dose at present for the management of PE is ten milligrams of Paxil daily or twenty-five milligrams of Zoloft daily for two weeks straight as a loading dose followed by use on an as-needed basis. In my experience, combining Paxil with some of the PDE-5 inhibitors has an even higher success rate.

Recently, a medicine called Priligy (dapoxetine) was developed specifically for the management of PE. It is rapidly absorbed and increases ejaculatory delay from the first dose and is administered on an as-needed basis. Although Priligy is still waiting for approval by the FDA, its future looks promising in resolving the problem of premature ejaculation.

A History of Treating PE

Prior to 1990, when urologists began trying the off-label use of a number of these antidepressants to treat PE, the problem was viewed as a psychological impasse, and not a physical failure, and psychotherapy was the treatment of choice. In the 1940s, clinicians proposed the stop-start technique, also known as the Masters and Johnson method. This involves stopping intercourse when the man perceives ejaculatory inevitability, allowing it to subside, and then resuming intercourse, repeating this cycle until both partners are satisfied. In the late 1960s, sexual therapists developed a model that included individual and joint therapy sessions, along with behavioral techniques such as the sensate focus and the squeeze technique (discussed more thoroughly in chapter 15). I recommend to my patients that they first try these nonpharmacological self-help techniques. If they still report difficulty in delaying ejaculation, I may recommend one of the off-label uses of SSRIs or PDE-5 inhibitors, but all men should realize that premature ejaculation should be viewed as simply another challenge in the quest to becoming a superpotent man. I have known many superpotent men who overcame PE and have gone on to have healthy and long-lasting intimate relationships. The only question is whether you are willing to over*come* what makes you *come* too quickly.

Chapter 5

Prostatic and Other Urologic Diseases

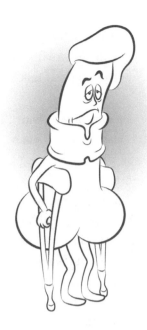

The term *urologic diseases*, when applied to men, refers to certain conditions of the urinary and reproductive systems. Several common urologic conditions and diseases are discussed below.

BPH: Don't Panic!

As if getting old is not difficult enough, a significant number of aging men develop a frustrating and sometimes painful condition known as benign enlargement of the prostate or benign prostate hypertrophy (BPH), which creates an obstruction to the flow of urine. BPH is present in more than half of all men over the age of fifty. It is *not* related to prostate cancer. BPH is a benign condition that causes discomfort, incomplete bladder emptying, frequent urination (particularly at night), and a weak urinary flow. While it carries symptoms that affect the quality of daily life, it is not lethal.

BPH can best be described by this anecdote:

> A patient walks into a urologist's office and sits down
> in the consultation room. The doctor, who has a stutter,

61

> asks the patient, "What is is is is wr-wr-wr-wrong wi-wi
> with ya-ya-you?" The patient answers, "Well, Doc, I piss
> the way you talk."

The case of a patient I'll call Jerry helps shed light on the issues related to prostate disease. Jerry was a sixty-six-year-old chemistry professor who was waking up three or four times a night to urinate. His urine flow was slow and irregular. He felt a sensation of incomplete bladder emptying. All these complaints suggested he might be suffering from a benign enlargement of his prostate.

You can think of the prostate as a collar or a doughnut surrounding the neck of the bladder, and the bladder as an upside-down balloon. As a man gets older, the collar or doughnut (prostate) tends to get bigger and the doughnut hole smaller. The shrinking hole pinches the neck of the bladder, making urination more difficult. This causes the bladder to work harder to empty itself. This phenomenon can lead to other symptoms besides those Jerry reported, including blood in the urine, a dribbling urinary stream, painful urination, occasional incontinence, and sometimes pain in the lower back, pelvis, or lower abdomen.

I took a detailed medical history, after which I performed a digital rectal examination (DRE) with my "educated" gloved finger. I assessed the size and consistency of his prostate and then used a funnel-like device that measures the urinary flow rate. I performed a bladder scan to assess Jerry's residual urine, trying to determine his ability to completely or incompletely empty his bladder. Next, I performed a quick prostatic ultrasound, a test that projects sound waves through the prostate to search for signs of cancer. The results were negative.

Finally, I used a cystoscope, a fiberoptic instrument that is inserted directly into the urinary channel. With the help of various lenses, doctors can examine the entire length of the urethra, looking directly at the prostate and then into the bladder in order to check for tumors, polyps, stones, and other causes of irritation. In addition, the cystoscope allows for assessment of the size and degree of prostatic obstruction. The procedure when skillfully performed is relatively painless and is done in the office in about thirty seconds.

Following this complete examination, I concluded that Jerry's prostate was enlarged to the point where damage might eventually be done to his bladder or his kidneys and recommended aggressive treatment in the form of a surgical procedure known as a prostatectomy.

Jerry panicked, not because he did not trust me to perform the surgery (which I had done successfully on thousands of patients, including Jerry's older brother *and* his uncle), but because he thought that the operation would render him a penis weakling. Jerry's reaction is so common, and I must state emphatically that prostatectomy, when done for benign disease, does not cause impotence or any loss of penis power!

Alternatives to a Prostatectomy

Over the past several years, many effective, noninvasive, and safe nonsurgical treatments for BPH have been developed. In the realm of medication, two drugs in particular act directly to stop and even reverse enlargement of the prostate gland. The older of these two, Proscar (finasteride), reduces a potent androgen (the male hormone equivalent to the female estrogen) that is responsible for the enlargement of the prostate. Although this drug works slowly over time, most urologists note a reduction in both the overall size of the prostate and the severity of obstructive symptoms. The only drawback is that since it reduces the blood concentration of a potent androgen, it can, on occasion, affect the patient's libido.

A newer drug, Avodart (dutasteride), also improves the symptoms of prostatic enlargement. This drug reduces the androgen that is responsible for prostatic enlargement and reduces the risk of acute urinary retention and the need for surgery. Over the course of many months, my patients have reported impressive reductions in the symptoms of prostatic obstruction with the use of Avodart, and also minimal side effects.

I often prescribe three other drugs along with Avodart or Proscar that operate by an entirely different mechanism of action. These drugs (Flomax, Rapaflo, and Uroxatral) are known pharmacologically as alpha-blockers. When men get older, the prostate (the doughnut around the neck of the bladder) gets bigger, and the hole in it gets smaller. The alpha-blockers make the hole bigger, allowing a more complete emptying of the bladder. When alpha-blockers are taken at the same time as anti-androgens (Proscar or Avodart), they work synergistically, and symptoms of benign enlargement of the prostate can often be dramatically improved.

Turn Up the Heat: TUMT

Not all men with symptoms of BPH respond well to these drugs. In some cases, the degree of prostatic obstruction is so pronounced that a more aggressive approach is needed, but even these more serious cases can be handled without surgery. A nonsurgical treatment for BPH was developed a number of years ago known as dose-optimized thermal (DOT) therapy or transurethral microwave therapy (TUMT). This involves the use of heat in the form of microwaves. DOT or TUMT delivers a specific "best dose" of heat to a patient's prostate, reducing the obstructive element and allowing maximum relief of symptoms with the fewest side effects.

To be certain a patient is a good candidate for thermal therapy and the DOT or TUMT procedure, I first perform a thorough evaluation with the cystoscope, as well as with a prostate ultrasound, used to assess both the size of the prostate and the degree of obstruction. If the degree of prostatic obstruction is significant, the patient is given a return appointment for the in-office DOT or TUMT treatment, which takes about forty-five minutes. The heat is applied through a small, flexible catheter that is inserted into the penis. There is no cutting or incision and minimal discomfort. This special catheter delivers the exact amount of heat needed to destroy the obstructive prostate tissue and usually results in the long-lasting relief of all symptoms of BPH. In my clinical experience, no men have had problems with erection or ejaculation as a result of the DOT or TUMT treatment.

As with any medical treatment, the microwave therapy is not for everyone.

Call the Roto-Rooter Man

In some cases, the large size of the prostate or the severe degree of bladder outlet obstruction requires a more aggressive approach. With the advent of new medical technology, prostate operations for benign disease do not even require a surgical incision but can be done through the penis—a transurethral prostatectomy (TURP). This is a technique that uses either laser ablation (GreenLight laser) or electrocauterization. Some of my patients have dubbed this the Roto-Rooter technique. Almost all benign prostatic obstruction can be cured in this manner.

As with the standard cystoscope, the TURP or GreenLight laser involves entering the prostate through the urinary channel. The ingenious laser beam, or cutting and coagulating device, is inserted, enabling the doctor to core out the obstruction (the compressed hole in the doughnut). This method is quick, is relatively painless, and is by far the simplest and safest nonincisive surgical method of relieving prostate obstruction. In most cases, patients do not need to be hospitalized, but even if they do, they usually return home within twenty-four hours. Recovery is painless and brief. Unlike the old procedure, which required an abdominal incision, this new method has a low risk of postoperative penis weakness. As one of my patients so eloquently told me, the procedure resulted in his "pissing like a racehorse."

If, like Jerry, you are a superpotent man, and you were capable of getting firm erections *before* a TURP (done with or without a laser), you will be just as potent after the procedure. Your penis power may even be enhanced, not because of what the surgery does to your genitals, but because reversing the effects of prostate enlargement—distended bladder, abdominal bloating, pelvic pain, and rectal pressure—can improve your general well-being, and with it your sexuality.

If you suffer from an enlarged prostate and your physician determines that all conservative treatment options have been exhausted, do not hesitate to correct a prostate problem with these routine transurethral procedures. The prostate is a secondary sex organ, not directly responsible for erection or ejaculation. One possible side effect of a TURP (with *or* without laser ablation) must, however, be mentioned:

retrograde ejaculation. In about 30 percent of post-TURP patients, little or no semen comes out of the penis during ejaculation. Instead, when the patient climaxes, semen is ejaculated *backward* into the bladder. While this may sound alarming, retrograde ejaculation is harmless. The ejaculate is evacuated with the next passage of urine. Naturally, retrograde ejaculation presents an obstacle to fertility and thus is more disturbing psychologically than it is medically. It does not affect the sensation of orgasm.

A few of my patients have told me that backward ejaculation "makes sex about 10 percent less fun." I suspect that the minor reduction in enjoyment is because men feel strange about this new process, but most get used to it and even laugh about the fact that their partners find sex far less messy than it was in the old days.

Prostate Cancer

Other diseases that afflict the genitourinary system carry with them a much greater threat, both to life and to penis power. I refer principally to cancer.

Prostate cancer is one of the most serious health problems in the global community. It is the most common male malignancy and has touched almost every family. Prostate cancer is the second most common cause of death from all neoplasms (tumors).

Recently, the rate of prostate cancer among men caught up to that of lung cancer. More than two hundred thousand cases are detected each year in the United States alone. About one in every six men in the United States will develop the disease during his lifetime. The rate of incidence increases dramatically with age. Almost 60 percent of those afflicted are over the age of sixty-five.[1]

In the last thirty years, there has been a dramatic increase in the number of cases of prostate cancer detected each year. This is due to the rising median age of our population, as well as our ability to detect the tumor at an earlier and more curable stage. With the PSA (prostatic specific antigen) blood-screening test, transrectal prostate ultrasonography, and heightened public awareness, the increase in the number of cases is being met with an increase in effective treatment. When patients learn they have prostate cancer, they often lament, "You might as well cut off my penis!" In almost all cases, their fear of impotence is totally unwarranted.

Treatment depends on a number of factors, including physical condition and the type and stage of the cancer cells at the time of diagnosis. In many cases, the recommended treatment is a total nerve-sparing prostatectomy. This entails surgically removing the *entire* prostate gland as opposed to removing only the portion that obstructs urine flow. This is done by creating only a coin-sized incision. A laparoscope (a fiberoptic microcamera instrument) and the da Vinci robot, a revolutionary computerized surgical device, assist in the procedure by providing magnification and enhanced dexterity to the surgical hand. With the advent of the da Vinci technology in 1999, the surgical approach to treating prostate cancer took a giant leap forward.[2]

Because the prostate is a secondary sexual organ, your penis can perform perfectly well without it. The old surgical cure for prostate cancer left 60 to 80 percent of patients impotent since surgery damaged the vital nerve bundles that make erection possible. Today, approximately 80 percent of our patients emerge from their recuperation with their full penis power intact. The other 20 percent get help with the aid of oral erectile dysfunction drugs, injection therapy (prostaglandin-E1), or occasionally a penile prosthesis.

The most essential aspect of ensuring the preservation of normal life expectancy and a high quality of life is the early diagnosis and prompt treatment of the prostate cancer, and the approach to treatment varies and is heavily dependent on the extent of the prostate cancer at the time of diagnosis. The prognosis is best in organ-confined disease (meaning a cancer that has not yet spread to other parts of the body). Utilizing the laparoscope with the da Vinci robot avoids severing any muscle tissue, which is the key reason this surgical procedure has had especially good results with regard to restoring continence (urine control) and maintaining erectile function. Based on the improved understanding of the anatomy of the neurovascular bundle (the packet of nerves and blood vessels that run like railroad tracks, on both sides of the prostate and are essential for erectile function) and the continence mechanism, the newest surgical techniques have made prostate surgery safe and effective.

Despite the new and improved techniques, surgery is suitable only for those patients whose cancer is completely confined to the prostate gland without any evidence of extension beyond the capsule (outer shell) of the prostate or into the adjacent lymph nodes.

The key to early diagnosis and potential cure is a yearly digital rectal examination by a qualified examiner, a PSA blood test, and an ultrasonic-guided prostate biopsy, if needed. Once the diagnosis of prostate cancer is made, the key to treatment is based upon the underlying stage of the disease. Differentiating between prostate cancer that is entirely confined to the prostate gland and prostate cancer that has spread beyond the margins of the gland is essential.

The development of magnetic resonance imaging (MRI) has revolutionized prostatic imaging and the staging of the disease. For the first time, we can visualize the internal architecture of the prostate gland prior to surgery. With this sophisticated and precise ability to observe the position and extent of a tumor, we can map all the tissue around the prostate; we can view neurovascular bundles, seminal vesicles, venous complexes, and regional lymph nodes.

In properly selected patients, surgery can provide a disease-free survival rate of up to thirty years, comparable to the expected survival rate of similarly aged healthy men. To determine which patients are candidates for surgery, the disease's natural history (that is, its biological aggressiveness) needs to be weighed against the patient's life expectancy. Life expectancy is based on risk factors referred to as comorbidities: heart disease, hypertension, diabetes, obesity, and family history.

As a general rule, if a patient has organ-confined prostate cancer and, in my judgment, his life expectancy is ten years or greater based on actuarial statistics, the patient is an excellent candidate to have his cancer surgically removed utilizing the laparoscopic robotic technique. My first obligation as a urologic surgeon is to do the best cancer operation I can for the patient. If the prostate tumor has extended to the adjacent nerve bundle, I will cut the nerve bundle to remove the malignant tissue. Most patients would agree that a surgeon's primary responsibility is to effectively obliterate the cancer. Preserving life sometimes requires a sacrifice of penis power. Surgeons do everything possible to avoid that contingency, but when it is absolutely necessary, we make the choice knowing that we can take further steps later to help restore penis power.

Since most cancers, particularly those diagnosed at an early stage in older men, are slow growing, there has been some controversy about treatment. Published data has examined "watchful waiting" as a legitimate treatment option. The patient must be sufficiently informed about the available modalities of treatment so that he can express his treatment preferences. Decision making must be shared between a knowledgeable physician and the patient.

The other modalities of treatment that should be considered when the patient is deemed curable include pinpoint IMRT (intensity-modulated radiation therapy) and the implantation of radioactive seeds, or a combination of both. Though modern radiation therapy and the "seeds" have been very effective, the disease-free survival rate of patients treated with the radiation option is not as good as for those treated with surgery if the tumor is confined to the prostate.

Recently, a number of treatment options have been developed that may soon find their way into clinical practice. The most promising is high intensity focused ultrasonography (HIFU), an alternative treatment option for localized prostate cancer. It has been used in Europe for several years and was recently approved for limited use in the United States by the FDA. It employs a transrectal ultrasonically powered probe that generates heat to selectively treat those focal areas of the prostate that are involved with biopsy-proven cancer. The *theoretical* advantages of this treatment are clear:

- The entire prostate need not be treated.
- The risk of damaging the nerves controlling erectile function is decreased, so post-treatment impotence is less of a concern.
- Since the entire prostate is not treated and the urinary sphincter is untouched, post-treatment incontinence is rare.

The use of HIFU as a modality for treating the entire prostate has proven to be problematic because of the increased risk of rectal injuries. However, the technique has been used for "salvage" treatment—treatment of prostate cancer that recurred, particularly after radiation treatment (either external beam radiation or radioactive seed implantation or both).

As of this writing, there is not enough long-term data to evaluate the technique's effectiveness and side effects. So at the present time, I can only recommend it as an *alternative* treatment. Only time will tell if it becomes mainstream.

Up to this point, we have restricted discussion to a cancer that is confined to the prostate alone. There is still much hope for curing more advanced prostate cancers, including cancers that have spread beyond the confines of the prostate gland. Even though patients in this category are not candidates for surgical removal of the tumor, well-established treatment with hormonal manipulation, radiation, and chemotherapy (often in combination) offers excellent results.

Patients must educate themselves. Patient awareness not only makes my job easier but also allows the patient to assume a proactive and participatory role in the treatment process. Published data has shown that screening using the PSA blood test in conjunction with a standard digital rectal examination doubles the detection rate of early prostate cancer.

You cannot actually *prevent* prostate cancer—not by diet or activity, nor even by picking your parents wisely. We must turn to early diagnosis to beat the deadly potential of this disease. Thousands of patients in my clinical practice have lived long and productive lives with prostate cancer. With a thorough examination, the ability to make a timely diagnosis is nearly 100 percent. If the diagnosis is made early enough to allow the maximum effective treatment, life after prostate cancer surgery or other treatment can be rich and rewarding, allowing a man to be continent, sexually active, and vigorous in all areas of his life.

A similar situation exists for other cancers in the genitourinary tract, including testicular cancer.

Testicular Cancer

Testicular cancer, which affects mainly younger men, is relatively rare. This form of cancer is the most easily treated of all tumors in the genitourinary system. Just twenty-five years ago, more than 90 percent of patients with certain types of testicular cancer did not survive five years. Now, a majority of cases are curable.

Consider the story of Olympic gold-medal winner Scott Hamilton. While on tour with Stars on Ice in 1997, he was diagnosed with testicular cancer that had spread to his abdomen. After undergoing aggressive chemotherapy and removal of the cancerous testicle, he was completely cured. He returned to the ice within months of his diagnosis. Without the amazing advancements of modern medicine, this would not have been possible.

In most cases where surgery is required for testicular cancer, we remove one of the two testes. Cancer rarely affects both at the same time. The surviving gonad will compensate by producing additional testosterone. Even if we have to remove both testes, we can preserve normal masculine functioning with testosterone injections, patches, or topical gels. These treatments maintain normal levels of circulating serum testosterone.

Kidney Transplants

Kidney failure also deserves discussion. The main reasons for kidney failure include uncontrolled diabetes, cardiovascular diseases such as hypertension or arteriosclerosis, chronic kidney infections, and viral diseases. For some patients who undergo kidney transplants, the penis power prognosis is not so good. Most patients who require kidney transplants have one or more of these severe underlying disorders, many of which have a negative effect on erectile function and libido.

While most of my patients with only *one* kidney transplant often maintain penis power, those forced to undergo a second transplant typically report erection failure afterward. This happens because the blood supply that ordinarily serves the penis is "borrowed" for the newly transplanted kidney. Many patients with kidney failure are on dialysis while they wait for an organ suitable for transplantation. During that phase, libido and sexual function usually decline. In addition, more than half of my patients on chronic dialysis develop penis weakness based on the effects of their underlying disease, certain endocrine complications, and psychological despair.

When a good matching kidney is found and the transplant is successful, a patient can expect to return to a healthy sex life with an abundance of penis power. This is especially true for those patients who have a good handle on their underlying disease. If you suffer from diabetes, hypertension, or other cardiovascular disorders, the best approach is to ensure meticulous supervision of your illness and do everything in your power to improve your health by seeking medical help and following the advice of your doctors.

The Good News

It's important to note that the disorders discussed in this chapter are not a death sentence to penis power. Only *some* diabetics, *some* men with nerve disease, *some* hypertensives, and *some* cancer patients become impotent. These conditions might produce only a *partial* loss of penis power, or none at all. In many cases, the impact on penis power can be reversed with medical treatment or lifestyle changes. Even with bona fide organic disorders, a significant portion of penis weakness is psychological. When these patients learn that organic disorders can cause erection problems, the thought alone weakens penis power in all but the most self-confident men.

As with any setback, attitude is vital. A sick man with a positive mind-set will find ways to continue enjoying his sexuality to the maximum extent possible. A man with a superpotent attitude can retain his penis power regardless of his physical condition, even if he has to stretch his imagination and alter his sex habits.

Ultimately, where there is penis power, there is a way.

Chapter 6

Blue Pills and Other Medical Cures for Erectile Dysfunction

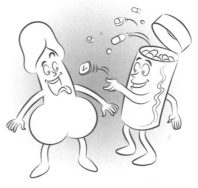

Modern technology has enabled medical professionals to help men with superpotent attitudes to function as normally as possible, even those with irreversible organic impotence. Three-quarters of what we now do could not have been done even ten years ago. Below are some options.

Blue Magic: The Saga of "the Pills" for Men

No single development over the past thirty years has changed the landscape of men's health as dramatically as the recent widespread use of erectile dysfunction medication. Urologists refer to these as the pills.

Prior to 1997, the only options for the treatment of impotence involved "body-shop" mechanics. Methods included the surgical implantation of a penile prosthesis (similar to a breast implant) and the use of a vacuum erectile device (VED), which has the look of a toy and is often advertised in the back of men's magazines. The last days of the twentieth century heralded the arrival of the "magic blue pill." Viagra, by Pfizer, revolutionized the treatment of erectile dysfunction.

The drug, known as a PDE-5 inhibitor, was discovered serendipitously, first developed as a vasodilator in the treatment of hypertension and coronary artery disease. Initial clinical studies showed that the drug was not very effective for this purpose. The manufacturer asked for the male patients involved in the study to return the drug. To the manufacturer's surprise, few did, and when asked why, patients replied that after taking the drug, they obtained the kind of firm erections they remembered only from their youth. The revolution began.

Currently, five erectile dysfunction drugs are on the market. Viagra, the first to be introduced commercially, was followed by Cialis, whose effects last longer. Levitra, which has a profile similar to that of Viagra, followed. Staxyn and Stendra are the most recently approved drugs. All five operate in a similar way.

To obtain a proper erection, the pills must be taken approximately thirty to sixty minutes before sexual activity. The penis still must be stimulated, either physically or psychologically. The main chemical at work in all these drugs is a PDE-5 inhibitor that boosts the enzyme that relaxes the smooth muscle cells inside the penis. Sexual excitement combined with the drug enables the arteries in the penis to widen and the spaces in the erectile chambers to fill with blood. As the veins in the penis expand, they trap blood in the penis for a prolonged period. These drugs seem to be remarkably effective in patients who have an organic (biological) reason for their impotence. However, they seem to exert little impact on men who are getting adequate erections but are using them as "performance-enhancing" drugs.

It's Not Candy

Understanding that these pills are not aphrodisiacs or sexual cure-alls is important. They will not work in the absence of desire, nor will they make an erection any harder or longer than what was normal for a man before he began experiencing erectile dysfunction. Almost all aspects of sexuality (attraction, desire, arousal, and orgasm) remain 99 percent between the ears. When the brain is stimulated by sexual fantasies or touch, it sends a signal through the nervous system directly to the penis. The signal releases nitric oxide (commonly known as laughing gas and historically used by dentists for anesthesia) in the penis. The release of nitric oxide causes the relaxation of the smooth muscles within the penis and allows blood to flow freely into the spongy tissue. This produces a firm erection.

At the same time, the veins that take blood out of the penis constrict. This constriction keeps the blood trapped in the spongy tissue until the sex act is completed. These pills inhibit the chemical that breaks down nitric oxide. It is this breakdown process that causes loss of an erection. By blocking the breakdown, these drugs create a longer period of smooth muscle relaxation in the penis, allowing the penis to stay erect for longer.

The pills are not "desire" drugs. They are "capacity" drugs, giving a man the *capacity* to exercise his sexual potential.

Lovemaking, and sex in general, involves intimacy, sensuality, and an emotional connection based on respect and caring, and these drugs are designed to help individuals revive and maintain the sexual aspects of a healthy relationship. Couples with problems in their interpersonal relationship should not turn to drugs as a quick fix or as a substitute for resolving conflicts. Communication and discussion are more valuable than any medicine.

Use with Caution

A partner with erectile dysfunction is often angry, depressed, and frustrated. This is especially true if the couple has not had sex in a long time. For this reason, if the pill is effective, major psychological and physical adjustments must be made in the sexual perspectives and practices of both partners. The good news is that each of these pills takes about thirty minutes to work, allowing time for intimacy, tenderness, and foreplay.

On the other hand, if a man takes the pill without informing his partner, gets a firm erection in about thirty minutes, and assaults his partner, his actions are certain to weaken the relationship. An impotent man newly empowered by the effects of the powerful pill must communicate if he hopes to have a meaningful ongoing sexual relationship with his partner.

Prior to the introduction of the pills, it was my clinical observation that the men who suffered from erectile dysfunction would usually shy away from any verbal or physical expression of sexual desire, fearing raising false hopes in their partners. Their partners, in turn, avoided sex out of fear of inducing guilt. If a couple wants their sexual interaction to be anything more than physical, both partners need to make significant psychological and emotional adjustments in the way they view their sex lives. I have witnessed couples who had problems within their interpersonal relationship who did not address deeper issues prior to swallowing the pill, and in all cases, the benefits generated by the ability to perform failed to deal with the emotional aspects of intercourse.

My advice to all of my patients is, if you are considering taking one of these powerful pills, take the time to discuss the ways in which this medication will change the nature of your relationship. Resolve underlying frustrations and grievances so that the bedroom does not become an escape from the realities of a frustrated relationship. If you are anxious and imprudent and rush through any discussion of the deeper implications of a renewed sex life, this could result in conflicts that strain your relationship. Through patience, openness, and mutual understanding, both partners can ultimately receive the wonderful benefits of these pills.

You Are Not Alone

According to the National Institutes of Health (NIH), up to thirty million men in the United States, half of whom are under the age of sixty-five, suffer from some form of erectile dysfunction.[1] It affects more than one in four men ages fifty to fifty-nine and about one in two men over the age of sixty.[2] Data compiled shows that Viagra is effective in about 85 percent of all patients with pure psychological impotence.[3] It is effective in slightly more than 70 percent of men whose inadequate erections have an organic cause—including neurological disorders, poor blood supply (caused by vascular diseases), or diabetes—or are a consequence of prostatic surgery.[4]

These medications are most effective in patients whose erectile dysfunction has resulted from spinal injuries or from surgery for prostate cancer. Their enormous appeal is their ease of use. They can be taken orally and discreetly many hours prior to the desired time for erection. Unlike the injectable medications (prostaglandin-E1, Caverject), which produce an erection regardless of stimulation, the individual *must* be sexually stimulated in order for these pills to work.

These are prescription medications and should not be taken without a thorough evaluation by a competent urologist or other qualified physician. Impotence is often an early indicator of a potentially serious underlying vascular or endocrine disease, and taking any of these drugs without a full medical evaluation could complicate these conditions to a life-threatening degree. If a patient with erectile dysfunction has silent, undiagnosed coronary heart disease and takes any of these drugs, he could suffer a fatal heart attack while having intercourse.

Though all these pills are relatively safe and carry minimal side effects, they are still potent. Even though they can cure a significant life-*altering* condition, the underlying cause of the dysfunction can be a life-*threatening* condition. These drugs should never be used in patients who are taking any form of nitrates, such as nitroglycerin, organic nitrates, or "poppers" (amyl nitrates), drugs commonly used in patients with coronary artery disease. The most significant side effects are minor and include headaches, facial flushing, nonspecific back pain, alteration in perception of the color blue, and heartburn. In my practice, very few men discontinue use of the pills due to these side effects.

When a patient comes to me in distress about penis failure, I first reassure him that everything will be all right. Once we define the cause of the dysfunction, we can assign an appropriate treatment option. With the pills, we start with the lowest prescribable dose (Viagra, twenty-five milligrams; Cialis, Levitra, and Staxyn, ten milligrams; and Stendra, fifty milligrams) and slowly move up to the maximum prescribable dose if needed. If the oral medications are not suitable or do not work, other corrective treatments might be more beneficial, including injection therapy, an intra-urethral suppository (Muse), hormonal therapy, or in some cases a surgical prosthesis.

These pills have worked *magic* for millions of men, but they may not help all men with impotence. All these drugs have the ability to dilate blood vessels and when taken in combination with certain other drugs, particularly nitroglycerin, may cause a sudden drop in blood pressure. Sometimes this may lead to death. The indiscriminate use of these pills can mask serious underlying medical conditions. Please heed my advice: see a doctor before taking any of these drugs!

Do Not Let the Hype Fool You

The long-term effects of continuous and large doses of Viagra, Cialis, Levitra, Staxyn, or Stendra, especially in men taking them for marginal reasons, remain unknown. I have found that the media often create an ideal of perfect sexuality, and many people believe they have to live up to certain standards of sexual behavior dictated by unrealistic portrayals. Within this idealized realm, anyone who is less than a herculean lover is unacceptable. However, in my clinical experience, most women *do not* want their partners erect for twelve hours. The advertised phrase for Cialis—"If your erection lasts longer than four hours, call your doctor"—sounds at first like the primal rallying cry for all superpotent men. In fact, most women are more than satisfied with ten to fifteen minutes of intercourse surrounded by tenderness and expressions of intimacy. Most women outright reject an erection marathon.

I have found that gay and bisexual men are four times more likely than heterosexual men to use the drugs for marginal or recreational reasons. They also are more inclined to view a longstanding erection as a badge of honor. Unfortunately, use of the pills in the gay community is often associated with the abuse of narcotics, especially at sex parties that include the use of crystal methamphetamine, cocaine, ecstasy, or ketamine. The combination of these drugs with the pills can and does result in serious cardiac or neurological problems, or both, and is also associated with the spread of sexually transmitted diseases, including HIV and AIDS.

Men taking medication for HIV infections not only are more likely to suffer from erectile dysfunction but also are much more *sensitive* to the effects of the oral medication. Certain protease inhibitors, the mainstay of treatment for HIV-positive patients, can markedly increase the blood concentration of oral erectile dysfunction drugs and may result in the magnification of both the effectiveness of these drugs and their potential side effects. Therefore, in HIV patients taking these drugs, the smallest possible dose of the PDE-5 inhibitors must be used to achieve adequate performance levels and safety margins that are acceptable.

From Pills to Pellets: The Muse System

Another relatively new drug commonly employed to correct erectile dysfunction utilizes an effective chemical known as alprostadil, or prostaglandin-E1 (PGE-1). In the past, this active chemical was only available for direct injection into the penis using either the Caverject or Edex system.

Many of my patients find the thought of injecting a tiny needle into the base of the penis unpleasant, painful, inconvenient, and in many cases impossible to master. Luckily, a more advanced delivery system is available that uses a drug marketed as Muse. This system also uses PGE-1, but employs it with a new and unique application system, an intra-urethral suppository.

With this system, the drug is delivered by very carefully inserting a small, soft pellet into the tip of the penis, where it comes in contact with the urethral mucosa (urinary channel). The pellet dissolves almost immediately. The drug is promptly absorbed into the bloodstream, causing rapid dilation of the vessels in the penis, resulting in a firm erection. The side effects are minimal and might include minor urinary discomfort.

Muse is the only noninjectable delivery system for PGE-1 and should only be used in men who have had a failed response to Viagra, Cialis, Levitra, Staxyn, or Stendra. The Muse system usually produces an erection within five to ten minutes after application. Based on what we know so far, it is both safe and effective. For patients using Muse, I ask them to urinate first, then insert the applicator one inch into the tip of the penis. The patient then gently pushes a button on the top of the plastic applicator and an effective dose of Muse is delivered to the urethral membrane. We usually start with the lowest dose of Muse (125 or

250 micrograms) and increase as necessary. I recommend a maximum frequency of use of one system per twenty-four-hour period.

Muse appears to provide consistent effectiveness regardless of the underlying cause of erectile dysfunction. The most serious local side effect so far has been priapism, the medical term for a persistent and painful erection. The risk of this appears to be less than one-half of one percent.[5] I must emphasize the need for a physician to calculate the proper dosage of Muse.

As with all the drugs used for erectile dysfunction, my patients are delighted with their improved emotional well-being and the enhanced quality of their interpersonal relationships. In the properly selected patient, the Muse system is an excellent alternative for the treatment of erectile dysfunction.

Shooting It Up: Injectable Medication

When the normal circulatory events that result in a good, firm erection cannot take place due to a physical disorder, urologists can instead produce a perfectly functional *pharmacological* erection. Our preferred method is to inject a medication into the shaft of the penis. The main drug used is PGE-1 (the same chemical used in the Muse system). PGE-1 is a vasoactive drug that relaxes the smooth muscles in the walls of the penile arteries and increases blood flow into the corpora within the penile shaft through vessels that are commonly blocked by arteriosclerotic plaque. The results are dramatic! The penis becomes semierect within five to ten minutes and quite rigid in fifteen minutes. In most instances, it remains erect for thirty to fifty minutes. Significantly, the drugs have no effect on orgasm or ejaculation.

The safe use of the injectable medication began nearly three decades ago. We are still confident in the effectiveness of this treatment method. With the use of this technique, we have restored thousands of penis-weakened men to active, fulfilling sex lives. After assigning the proper drug and determining the precise dosage for each individual patient, we meticulously train the patient to inject himself. The system uses a tiny needle and a small syringe similar to those used by diabetics who self-inject insulin.

Once we are satisfied that the patient has mastered the technique, we instruct him to inject the medication prior to intercourse. The injection will produce automatic results; an erection will result even in an anesthetized patient. Interestingly, however, erotic stimulation *enhances* the effect of the medication. This occurs because stimulation increases the presence of the circulating neurotransmitters released by the brain when it is sexually aroused. These chemicals complement the dynamics of the drugs. By contrast, the lack of privacy in the doctor's office can *reduce* the effect. The good news is that the drugs tend to work better in the bedroom than in the examining room.

These drugs must not be used without strict medical supervision, and active follow-up is essential. Men with conditions such as varicose veins, a condition in which blood tends to pool in the limbs; blood disorders such as sickle cell anemia; and unstable cardiovascular disease with symptoms such as fainting spells should not use injectable drugs. Those who have limited dexterity or poor eyesight—both of which could lead to errors when preparing the syringe or injecting the medication—should also avoid them. Additionally, I am cautious about prescribing this method for patients whom I consider emotionally unstable. As with any drug, there is potential for misuse. In such cases, I strongly recommend psychological counseling.

One possible misuse of injectable drugs is to take them too often. One of my patients, an extremely wealthy man in his sixties who had had a history of superpotent activity, reacted with anger when a vascular condition rendered him physically impotent. He had just married a much younger, world-class beauty. I prescribed a "vasoactive cocktail," a combination of PGE-1 and papaverine. I determined the proper dosage, taught him how to self-inject, and instructed him to inject the medicine no more than once every other day. And off he went to spend time with his new wife on their yacht in the Mediterranean. When he returned to Los Angeles, he came in for a checkup and raved about the therapy. He said he was having the best sex he'd had in thirty-five years—three times a day, sometimes for hours at a time. He could not have been happier. I could not have been more alarmed.

I was concerned with the potential side effects of medically inducing erections six hours a day! If an erection lasts too long, the blood trapped in the penis does not drain, and this can result in priapism and permanent damage to the delicate sinusoids within the penis. This may lead to impotence so severe that not even injectable drugs can counteract it.

Priapism occurs very rarely, almost always after the misuse of medication, but when it does occur, we have to act quickly to avoid permanent damage. We instruct patients to phone us or the paramedics immediately if an erection lasts longer than four hours. We inject a Neo-Synephrine solution directly into the shaft of the penis to gradually reduce tumescence (erection). In many cases, we give patients an emergency syringe with a proper dose of Neo-Synephrine to be kept at home.

Other side effects that sometimes arise from injection therapy include dizziness, headaches, a metallic taste in the mouth, bruising or inflammation of the penis, tingling sensations, and swelling or angulation after the injection. Most of these local complications are minor and can be avoided if the patient follows our instructions to the letter.

Those instructions are rigorous, and informed consent is vital. My staff and I spend a great deal of time with the patient and his partner explaining the action of the drugs, the theory behind the therapy, the proper dosage and application, and the risks and possible side effects. Each patient is also given a packet of printed material to take home with him for further information.

One of the main considerations for the urologist is to determine the appropriate *combination* of drugs to be injected and their proper dosages. Not all men react the same way to a given dose of a vasoactive drug. We have to find the precise amount and create a custom-designed recipe for each patient. The ideal combination is exactly what is needed for that patient to achieve the goal—an erection that lasts thirty to forty-five minutes without side effects. The ideal dose varies depending on the underlying cause of the problem, the patient's state of mind, and the psychological environment in which he takes the drug.

Only after meticulously testing various doses in my office under controlled clinical conditions do I teach the patient to self-inject. And patient response varies. At one extreme are patients like the newly married, wealthy man who abused the privilege; at the other extreme are those who discontinue therapy either because they are afraid of complications, squeamish about injecting themselves, or turned off by the loss of spontaneity caused by having to stop and inject a drug into their penis. The majority of patients fall in the middle, grateful for the medical technology that enables them to have a satisfying sex life.

Surgical Procedures

At this point in time, we are unable to electively transplant a penis the way we can other organs. The penis has unique functions depending on a complex mix of nerve, blood, and hormonal variables, all hinging on delicate feedback mechanisms. With all my faith in modern science, I cannot imagine a time when impotent men will be rejuvenated by the surgical transplantation of real genitals. Even if the technology existed, we have so many simpler alternatives that I doubt it would ever be used.

Since many erection problems are caused by insufficient blood flow to the penis, medical science has naturally sought methods to reverse that problem. Studies so far have focused on ways to transfer blood from neighboring vessels to the deep arteries of the penis. These surgeries, still largely ineffective, have demonstrated some success in young men suffering from acute pelvic trauma. Due to the complex vascular anatomy of the penis, however, we have been unable to duplicate the success we have had with the treatment of other arterial disorders.

Experimental work has also been done on preventing venous leaks. An erection cannot be maintained unless the veins in the corpora hold in the blood. With modern diagnostic procedures, we can tell when blood is leaving the venous channels in abnormal amounts. Although work in this area is still in its infancy, surgery can be performed on selected patients to impede the backflow of blood from the penis and reverse the effects of a venous leak.

Pump It Up: Implants

The most common *surgical* procedure for impotence is the implantation of a penile prosthesis, a combination of ingenious design, technical proficiency, and durability that has made it possible to implant *directly* into the penis. In recent years, a variety of devices have been developed that enable surgeons to easily implant this device in an outpatient hospital setting, providing urologists with a permanent solution for thousands of organically impotent men who have the motivation to undergo surgery.

The implants allow for complete sexual satisfaction with a low rate of failure. At one point in the late 1980s, about thirty thousand prostheses were implanted each year around the world. Since the introduction of injectable medication (PGE-1), and more recently with the arrival of oral therapy, the number of prostheses has declined, though not as dramatically as one would think. This is largely due to increased promotion in the media for treatment of erectile dysfunction and the resultant creation of a larger pool of prospective surgical candidates.

There are basically two types of prostheses. The older variety is the so-called malleable implant, which consists of semirigid rods that are placed into the corpora. These implants make the penis rigid enough to successfully penetrate. The problem is that they do not change in length or girth, which means that the man has to walk around with a semifirm penis at all times. The device is flexible enough to bend into somewhat of a concealable shape, but the unnatural look may be a source of some embarrassment at the health club!

The second type of implant is the inflatable prosthesis consisting of two inflatable cylinders that are surgically implanted in the same corporal channels. It also includes a pump and a fluid-filled reservoir, usually implanted either within the scrotum or lower abdomen. When the patient desires an erection, he simply squeezes the pump several times. The fluid flows from the reservoir into the cylinders, which expand and swell, mimicking a natural erection. After intercourse, a release valve is simply pressed, and the fluid flows back into the reservoir, returning the cylinders to their empty state. The penis returns to its flaccid state. It is an ingenious design.

Because the inflatable model allows the user full control and leaves the penis looking relatively normal, my patients much prefer it. But it requires a slightly more extensive surgical procedure and has a higher rate of malfunction. Corrections require another surgical incision.

When I first began to implant the inflatable devices about twenty-five years ago, they were frequently plagued by mechanical failures requiring repeat surgeries. Recent improvements by manufacturers (particularly American Medical Systems) have been dramatic. The technology on the horizon promises to be even better. If inflatable prostheses continue to be profitable for manufacturers, more research and development dollars are likely to be allocated, leading to nonbreakable components that produce erections indistinguishable from the real deal.

A word about *my* mind-set: Before considering a patient for a prosthesis, I meticulously rule out all *correctable* medical conditions. Implantation is the treatment of last resort. When the decision is made, I inform the patient of the pros and cons of all available devices and still recommend the malleable device for many obese patients. If the penis is partially hidden by a protruding belly, its artificial firm appearance is not usually noticeable. With a slender man, however, the semirigid device stands out like the proverbial sore thumb.

Once chosen, the device is implanted, usually under regional anesthesia. One cylinder is placed in each corpora cavernosa. The surgical incision is small, buried unnoticeably in the scrotum. The procedure takes about thirty to forty-five minutes. Complications during and after surgery are extremely rare. Postoperative discomfort is relatively short-lived. Most bodies tolerate the implant almost as if it were made of flesh and blood.

Each prosthesis is customized for the individual, tailored to fit the precise length and width of the corpora. We cannot implant a prosthesis that is smaller, or the erections will have a floppy tip—the so-called SST deformity, named after the droopy nose of the Concorde supersonic transport plane. We also cannot implant a device that will make the penis longer, despite fantasies. In other words, after prosthesis, the functional penis, both erect and flaccid, will be the exact size it was before the implant.

For the Right Reasons

The ideal candidate for a prosthetic implant is someone with all the mental characteristics of a superpotent man, but one who is unable to achieve a satisfactory erection because of a real medical disorder. One of my patients was from a distant country with a vastly different culture from mine. One of the wealthiest men in the world, he had been married for thirty-five years to a woman he loved. He also had a concubine, an accepted custom in his society. For nearly twenty years, this man had fathered approximately one child each year. He then developed severe diabetes and was unable to have normal intercourse. After considering all the alternatives, he opted for a penile prosthesis. Ever since the surgery, he and his loving wife (and his concubine) have been grateful that the penis power that never left his heart was restored to the rest of his body.

For the Wrong Reasons

Another gentleman from the same part of the world represents the perfect example of the *wrong* reason to have a prosthesis. A member of a royal family, he came to my office at age forty-two for a urologic problem unrelated to sexuality. When I examined him, I noted that he had a primitive prosthetic device that had been implanted when he was only twenty-seven, when the devices available were crude. Visually, the result was grotesque.

I was curious *why* he chose to have the operation. He had no organic illness yet had chosen to endure the pain, embarrassment, and risk of having a crude plastic device implanted in his penis. His reasons were as repulsive as the prosthesis itself. He could afford anything in the world and owned all the homes, boats, planes, cars, and toys he could dream of. At the snap of his fingers, he could have an entourage of beautiful and willing women—and he snapped his fingers routinely, particularly when traveling outside his conservative nation. But the number and frequency of his erections were limited by physiology, so he *bought* himself an unlimited erection. His warped view of the penis and its power represents the best possible reason for *not* having a penile prosthesis.

A more typical candidate is the eighty-year-old retired man who wanted a prosthesis like the one that had restored his friend's sex life. Upon questioning, he revealed that he was in reasonably good health, but his marriage of more than forty years was unhappy, and he had few interests and low self-esteem. He had in effect given up on life. There was nothing wrong with his sexual apparatus that a renewed zest for life or a change of habit would not cure.

So why had I performed the operation on this man's friend? He was in his late seventies, had stayed involved in his business, and enjoyed a variety of recreational activities, and was a spirited widower involved with many younger girlfriends. In short, his penis power was not up to his penis demands due to a vascular problem that had necessitated bypass surgery. This man was a perfect candidate for an implant; his gloomy friend was not.

Mechanical Devices

For impotent men who seek an alternative to surgery or self-injection, several other devices are on the market. The most popular fall under the heading of "external vacuum therapy." Vacuum erectile devices (VED) produce erections by using suction, mimicking the physiology of oral sex. First, a plastic cylinder is placed over the penis. A vacuum is then created with a pump that draws blood into the penis, causing it to expand. When the penis becomes rigid enough for penetration—usually in a minute or two—the patient removes the cylinder and places a rubber band–like constricting device around the base of his penis that impedes venous outflow so that the erection can be maintained long enough for successful intercourse.

Vacuum erectile devices manufactured by reputable companies are safe and inexpensive with minimal risk of side effects. VEDs preclude the need for surgery, medication, or injections. On the other hand, they are awkward to handle and take a few minutes to assemble, thus reducing the pleasure and spontaneity of lovemaking. Rarely, the ring or rubber band used to impede the outflow of blood can inhibit ejaculation. Vacuum therapy is a reasonable alternative especially for those who suffer from *partial* loss of erection or who fear prosthetic implant surgery or injecting themselves with drugs, but professionally and personally, I highly recommend good old-fashioned oral sex, which has the same effect as a VED. In fact, it is even better because it is performed with the loving warmth of your partner's body.

Mechanical devices should be used under the supervision of a physician. Patients with blood disorders like sickle cell disease or clotting problems should not use these devices. Healthy men able to get satisfactory erections should not use a VED as a performance enhancement device. Such abuse is dangerous and would be the antithesis of penis power.

Aphrodisiacs and Other Substances

Nearly every culture in every period of history has a record of substances alleged to stimulate sexual desire and improve virility. These are derived mostly from plants and range from the infamous Spanish fly to complex combinations of Chinese herbs. Others include L-arginine, ginkgo, ashwagandha or "Indian ginseng," the Mexican herb damiana, and the plant extract called pygeum. Sadly, nearly an entire species of magnificent white rhinos has been slaughtered just to macerate their horns in the fruitless pursuit of penis power. Medical science has found no evidence that these aphrodisiacs work. They may have a placebo effect, but I have found no ingestible animal part or herbal substance that will cure penis weakness.

One herbal substance that may have some merits is *yohimbine*, derived from the bark of the yohimbe tree and considered an aphrodisiac by African cultures for hundreds of years. Dr. Christiaan Barnard, the eminent heart surgeon who pioneered human heart transplantation, used yohimbine on patients who developed impotence after surgery and reported satisfactory results in 75 percent of his cases. However, mainstream medicine does not embrace yohimbine therapy and its biochemical action is not understood. Dr. Barnard's original research was contaminated because yohimbine was used in combination with other drugs, primarily testosterone. So far, there is little reason to think that the bark of a tree can foster significant improvement in men with penis weakness.

Beware of the possible dangerous side effects of alternative treatments. One of my patients, in a dicey self-experiment, applied a nitroglycerin paste to the shaft of his penis. Because of its vasoactive profile, he concluded that it could increase penile blood flow. During sex, the substance was absorbed by his wife's vaginal mucosa, giving her severe headaches. The same might be true of the off-label use of minoxidil, which is marketed as an aid to hair growth in balding men. Because it also is a vasoactive substance, some have suggested that rubbing it on the penis might produce better erections (or even hair). I urge you to refrain from self-experiments with such products. There are plenty of proven alternatives.

Men all over the world spend billions of dollars every year in search of a magic elixir that can potentially cure penis weakness, and there are hundreds of hucksters hawking snake oils and cure-alls that have no verifiable scientific merit. As a physician, I have no reason to withhold legitimate, effective therapy for erectile dysfunction from my patients, but a scientific process exists for proving the effectiveness of any therapy. This consists of a double-blind, controlled, crossover study that justifies its use. I recommend my patients refrain from using any drug or substance that does not meet the strict standards of scientific inquiry.

The last years have seen magnificent medical advancements in the area of erectile dysfunction. I predict even more will be available to help with organic impotence in the near future. A small percentage of men with penis problems have true organic impotence; however, the vast majority of men have normal, perfectly capable penises served by well-functioning auxiliary organs. For millions, surgery, drugs, and mechanical aids have no place in their lives. The answer for them lies between their ears.

Chapter 7

Performance Anxiety: When It's All in Your Head

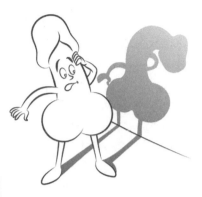

Steve, a thirty-nine-year-old lawyer, came to me wanting a complete urological workup; he was worried that something was wrong. He had met a great woman, and they had a terrific first date, but when she invited him in, as he told me, "one thing led to another and before I knew it we were in bed, and I couldn't . . . you know . . ."

I knew all right. I had heard it many times before from hysterical patients. Steve was terrified that something was wrong with his penis because he couldn't get an erection. I assured him this had nothing to do with physiology. He had gone through a bitter divorce and had been single for some time, and this date was the first time in years he had even kissed a woman other than his wife. He was just plain nervous—the excitement of meeting someone he liked and his eagerness to please her and prove himself a worthy bed partner conspired to create one of the greatest enemies of penis power: *performance anxiety*.

More penis weakness occurs the *first time* a man is with a partner than at any other time. When it happens, men feel so humiliated they sometimes find any excuse they can to avoid dating that person again. I have met men who, after several embarrassments, stayed away entirely from people who turned them on, in effect becoming celibate prisoners of penis performance anxiety.

This happens a lot with younger men. One patient, a college freshman named Cliff, was plagued by premature ejaculation and erection failure. In high school, misled by the bravado of his buddies, Cliff's earliest sexual experiences had been disasters. Because he was a handsome, rugged young man, he had no trouble finding dates, but when the sex did not work out, he was so mortified he never tried again with the same girl. His performance anxiety increased with every bad memory until he stopped dating altogether. In college, he created a fictitious out-of-town girlfriend. Cliff was as horny as a devil and tired of masturbating by the time he became convinced he needed medical help and got up the nerve to tell me about his "mechanical problem."

After I examined him, I explained he had no mechanical problem. "You have an attitude problem," I told him and assured him that his early sexual experiences were not unusual. Like getting back on a bicycle after you fall, you just have to try again—preferably with the same bicycle. I encouraged him to find a woman he liked and stay with her long enough to feel calm and trusting when they were in bed. "If things do not go right the first time, don't panic. If the woman has a heart, she'll understand. The next time you'll be much more relaxed." Within a short time, Cliff fell in love with a sweet, understanding woman and embarked on a steady, sexually satisfying relationship.

The first time with a new sexual partner can be exciting, but for some that excitement can lead to temporary penis weakness and can spiral into a disastrous pattern. It happens to young people like Cliff and to grown men like Steve who have been out of circulation. The same advice applies to both: take your time, be patient, stop pressuring yourself, and stop thinking you are inadequate. Find a partner who makes you feel comfortable and not threatened. Face the challenge with the courage it takes to overcome performance anxiety.

In addition, medical solutions are available. As an emergency measure, you can always carry a few Viagra or similar pills, but only as a last resort and after consulting with a urologist to be certain it is safe for you to use any of these strong prescription drugs (see chapter 6). But beware of the pills' "crutch effect" that can occur when you use a pill once and it works. Too often men conclude that they will never get an adequate erection without the drugs, but this does not address the real problem. Find the confidence to face your fears about sex and intimate relationships.

In my practice, performance anxiety is the leading cause of penis failure and is much more likely to happen to men who are with an unfamiliar partner or to men who feel pressured to measure up to some hypothetical sexual standard. Usually the cause is simple and obvious and can be fixed with a change of perspective or a change of circumstances. Losing an erection once in a while is as much a part of sex as booting a ground ball is to a shortstop or missing a target is to a marksman. If and when it happens, you have to be able to move on. Holding on to a memory of the failure will surely become the seed of future disappointments.

Accentuate the Positive

Whenever I meet men in leadership positions, I observe that they never think in terms of failure. They do not even use the term. They prefer *mistake* or *error* because the *f*-word implies a permanency they are unwilling to accept. Successful people focus on positive goals. Successful people put all their energy into the task at hand. They do not look back or make excuses or become intimidated by setbacks. If a particular situation does not go well, successful people analyze the situation and use the lessons learned to carve out future triumphs.

Of course, you have to learn the *right* lessons from setbacks. Cliff and Steve drew the *wrong* conclusions, coming away from their unsuccessful encounters with the idea that something was wrong with them. That is not the attitude that will fortify your penis power.

Management expert Warren Bennis coined a term that captures the superpotent attitude as it relates to performance anxiety: the Wallenda factor. He named it after the world-famous aerialist Karl Wallenda, the "Flying Wallenda." When Wallenda stepped out on the tightrope with nothing but air between him and the ground, he *never* thought of failure. He was seemingly impervious to the danger of falling, focusing his full attention on what he had to do at the moment. For fifty years, Wallenda was known as the most fearless and flawless aerial acrobat. Unfortunately, while Wallenda's career illustrates the importance of having the right attitude, his ultimate fate demonstrates what can happen if you do not.

In 1978, before walking a tightrope seventy-five feet above the ground, for some inexplicable reason, Wallenda, according to his wife, spent three months prior to this walk thinking of nothing but falling. "It was the first time he'd ever thought about that, and it seemed to me that he put all his energy into *not falling*, not into walking the tightrope."[1] For the first time in his career, he personally supervised the installation of the rope and checked to see that the guide wires were secure. Many believe that it was because of his preoccupation with falling that the great Wallenda fell to his death.

Metaphorically, this is exactly what Cliff and Steve and millions of other men do when they approach sex with their minds consumed by fear of failure: they end up defining their goal as "not embarrassing myself" rather than "having a good time." Having a negative perspective will prevent both you and your partner from extracting the maximum pleasure possible from a sexual encounter. Take a lesson from Wallenda: think about the task at hand, directing your attention completely to the sensual experience of making love.

Even the Strong Are Let Down Sometimes

When you begin to feel anxious or fearful, you are programming your mind for failure. Stop what you are doing, calm down, and remind yourself of what Franklin D. Roosevelt said at his inauguration: "There is nothing to fear but fear itself." What is the worst thing that could happen? You embarrass yourself? Only if you let yourself be embarrassed. These episodes happen to *every* man at some point in his sexual life so why should you be embarrassed? And what if you *are* embarrassed? How bad is that? Maintaining this positive point of view will keep you lighthearted, and your penis is likely to behave accordingly. Develop the ability to laugh at both yourself and that unpredictable appendage of yours, and you will both be winners. *Penis power is the power of positive thinking applied to your penis.*

I have had patients report back to me and say, "Well, Doc, I did what you said, and I was *still* nervous." Sometimes the fear is so deep rooted that you cannot bring yourself to believe in your own pep talk. As you fill your brain with positive thoughts, another part of your brain is snidely whispering, "Bullshit!" Still, keep those positive thoughts coming. Work at it relentlessly. In the long run, even the most cynical disbeliever will be convinced, and a positive attitude will result in reliable penis behavior.

Some men with a deeply rooted fear of penis failure do need more than a pep talk. Perhaps a prescription for an oral erectile dysfunction drug is just what is needed to break the vicious cycle, though I suggest such patients talk to a psychotherapist to explore deeper reasons for their anxieties. In most cases, low self-esteem and poor self-image affect not just sex but every aspect of these individuals' lives.

Unfortunately, compensating for low self-esteem is easier in business or sports than it is in bed. *Your penis never lies and is never fooled.* Your penis is a perfect reflection of your deepest thoughts and emotions. If you don't *think* you have a self-esteem problem but worry about your sexual performance, you may harbor some doubts about your masculinity. Self-doubt travels in a flash from the brain to the penis.

Consider the following:

- Do you constantly compare yourself to other men?
- When something minor goes wrong, do you scold yourself or call yourself insulting names?
- Do you judge yourself more harshly than you judge others?
- Do you find yourself trying hard to please other people?
- Do you strive to be liked by everyone?
- Are you overly sensitive to criticism?
- When you do something well, do you belittle your accomplishment?
- Do you have a strong need to prove yourself?

- When faced with a new challenge, do you immediately worry that you will not measure up?

If you answered yes to most of these questions, self-doubt is part of the problem, and your penis will pick up on that. If *you* do not think you are capable of good, solid penis performance, why should your penis act otherwise? If *you* do not think you deserve a fully satisfying sex life, why should your penis give you one? Work to raise your self-esteem. Look at all your positive accomplishments, at all your admirable traits. Examine the standards by which you measure yourself. If what you expect of yourself is based on standards imposed by other people, social institutions, or the media, you are not being true to yourself. Most importantly, recognize who you are and what your values are and do everything you can to live up to those personal standards and goals. *Set your own penis standards and then evaluate yourself with a fair and generous perspective.*

Do all this and your self-esteem will improve.

Lighten Up, Dude

Imagine, you are in bed with a sexy partner, whether your wife of thirty years or someone you just met. You start to worry that your penis will not get hard or that you might lose the erection that just popped up. Your first reaction might be to panic, worrying so much about your penis that tension builds. You get clumsy. You try to exert your willpower and forget about trying to excite your partner. You cannot appreciate, or even feel, your partner's loving kisses and strokes. One of two reactions is bound to happen next: your partner gets turned off and thinks she is doing something wrong, or your penis goes limp. It is usually both.

The minute you start to feel anxiety, stop what you are doing immediately and *tell* your partner you're nervous. Own up. Tell your partner you want so much to please her and bring her satisfaction and that her acceptance means a lot to you. Make sure she understands she is terrific and has not done anything wrong. Tell her the problem is all in *your* head and will surely go away. When it comes to your penis, honesty should be the *only* policy. Ninety-nine percent of the time, candor will improve the situation by diffusing tension. If you have a healthy relationship, your partner will appreciate your integrity and your vulnerability. She will probably reassure you, calm you down, and take the pressure off. If your partner instead gets angry, resentful, or demeaning, ask yourself if you are in bed with the right person.

And if you *do* fail to get an erection? If you *do* lose it at precisely the wrong moment? If you *do* ejaculate too quickly? Laugh it off! You're probably thinking, sure, that's easy for the doctor to say. But I mean it. I assure you that real men can and do laugh at their own penises or say funny phrases to their partners like, "Oh well, that rascal pulled a fast one on me." Expressed in your own words and style, lighthearted remarks should ease the tension and help your penis rise another day, or even the same day. Medically, I can practically guarantee it.

Your partner will be pleased to know that you are trying to improve your sexual ability and might have been thinking that something was wrong with *her*, that she was failing you. She might know you feel ashamed but not know what to say or do. Breaking the ice with a good laugh changes all that.

With all the unstated agendas, the physical clumsiness, and the childlike awkwardness, sex is just as suited for slapstick comedy as it is for fine art or soft-focus cinematography. Many people say there is no better turnon than a good, hearty laugh in bed, nothing sexier than a partner whose sense of humor is compatible with your own. Don't take your penis so seriously. That is how the trouble starts in the first place. And do not shy away from using your penis if it falls down on the job once or twice—or any number of times. In sex, as elsewhere, practice makes perfect.

I am reminded of a former patient I'll call Joe. Joe was a short man with a classic Napoleon complex. He had gone from one business to another, becoming fabulously successful in each one. A bachelor at forty, he talked so much about the women he dated I assumed he was having a healthy, varied sex life. To my astonishment, one day this human dynamo told me he was plagued by penis weakness. All of his accomplishments, it turned out, were a workaholic's futile attempts to gain the approval he never got from his father, a domineering man who raised his son to be emotionally fearful. Joe saw himself as worthless, and when alone with a woman, most of the time his performance was the equivalent of bankruptcy.

Joe had one great attribute: perseverance. He was a "never say it's over" kind of guy, and when he finally admitted his dissatisfaction with his penis performance, he delivered the same determination to the bedroom that he delivered to his work. A therapist helped him deal with his self-esteem, and I evaluated him urologically, assuring him he was fully capable of attaining penis power. Very soon after this boost in confidence and morale, his sexual relationships blossomed.

Another patient, Daniel, was a stark contrast. He also suffered from crippling self-doubt, but he expressed it in the opposite way. A classic *underachiever* in all aspects of his life, including sex, Daniel was an outstanding guitarist who had been a child prodigy; he was good looking and likeable, but low self-esteem prevented him from capitalizing on those traits. At twenty-nine, he eked out a living, and when he came to see me, he had not had a date in over a year. A series of disappointing experiences relegated sex and romance to pure fantasy. Unlike Joe, Daniel lacked the perseverance and the courage to expose himself to possible failure in order to conquer his fear.

Whenever I think of perseverance, I also think of a certain country lawyer who lost his job, lost an election for the state legislature, failed in private business, failed to land a nomination for the US Congress, and was twice defeated for the US Senate. He did all of this while persevering enough to earn some victories and ended up one of our most revered presidents. So the next time you are ready to give up on your penis, think of Abraham Lincoln.

There is a caveat: if you try *too* hard, you might make things worse. Some tasks succeed because of hard work and effort. Getting an erection is not one of them—the more you work at it, the less likely you are to succeed. It is analogous to falling asleep. Anyone who has ever tossed and turned with insomnia can tell you that the harder you *try* to sleep, the longer you stay awake.

It is what I call a Penis Paradox: *the harder you try, the softer it gets.* That was initially Joe's problem. He tried *so* hard to perform well that he could not relax enough to get an erection. Only when he learned to let go and simply enjoy what he was doing did nature take its course. From that point forward, his perseverance began to pay hefty dividends.

Just as your heart wants to beat, your lungs want to breathe, and your stomach wants to digest, your penis wants to get hard. Believe in your penis. Trust it. Give it every opportunity to do its job, but also give it the freedom you would give a trusted friend or colleague. Allow it to pursue its mission without you meddling or worrying. Just stay out of its way!

Don't Worry, Be Superpotent

Anxiety is the worst enemy of your penis, and I do not just mean anxiety about performance. If you are nervous about finances, the health of a loved one, your child's college application, or other troublesome aspects of adult life, your penis might let you down. Worry and fear cause wear and tear to the endocrine and nervous systems and cause blood vessels throughout the entire body to constrict. How could they *not* affect your penis?

Park your anxieties at the threshold to your bedroom. In fact, park them outside the house. Learn how to *compartmentalize your life* so that business is business, play is play, family is family, religion is religion, sex is sex. My most well-rounded, superpotent patients come by this skill naturally. No matter how much stress they're under at the office, they leave the stress when they leave the building. They never allow it to pollute their family lives or their sexual performance.

If you find it difficult to compartmentalize, work at it. If irrelevant, negative thoughts intrude on your penis performance, start by consciously sending those thoughts away and shifting your attention to the erotic sensations you are experiencing. Negative thinking is often just a *habit*. A psychologist colleague recommends a visualization exercise that can help you clear anxiety from your thoughts. In your mind's eye, see yourself gathering your troubles and placing them in a box. Then watch yourself seal the box and put it outside. People who view their feelings as forbidden territory may think this idea ridiculous, but if you are willing to try to make changes in your relationship with your body, such a technique can help get those worries out of the bedroom and give your penis permission to do what it likes to do most without interference. Acknowledging your emotions and being honest about what you are feeling is healthy. Talking about frustration and anger with someone you trust is helpful too. Accept things for what they are, do what you can to make them better, and then move on. These steps are essential in becoming confident in your penis performance. Emotional balance is a basic element in becoming a superpotent man.

I suggest cultivating what British philosopher and scholar Bertrand Russell called "the habit of thinking of things at the right time." The bedroom is not the place to plan next week's schedule, mentally rehearse a speech, or worry about tomorrow's board meeting. Russell wrote, "The wise man thinks about his troubles only when there is some purpose in doing so; at other times, he thinks about other things or, if it is night, about nothing at all."[2] Russell was referring to ways to sleep with greater ease, but apply the same thoughtlessness to penis activities, and you will be a superpotent man.

Exercise is a helpful way to burn off stress. You might find it easier to compartmentalize before you get intimate with your lover if you lift weights, run a few miles, or swim a few laps. Better yet, burn it off *in* bed. That's right—the best way I know of to get rid of stress is to have sex, which presents another Penis Paradox: stress can interfere with penis power, but exercising your penis power is a terrific way to eliminate stress.

I cannot count the number of superpotent men who have told me that their favorite antidote for their high-pressured professional lives is to hurry home to their partners. Sex is wonderful for clearing the mind, and it has fringe benefits that other physical activities cannot approach: sharing affection, experiencing intimacy, and feeling good about yourself. If you can learn to channel your frustration, anger, and worries into sexual energy, you can turn the tables on stress. Great performers use anxiety as an energizer and motivator, channeling it into their performances; that real emotional energy can make a performance spectacular—on the stage and in bed!

A patient who was a Hollywood talent agent came to me complaining of stress. His workday was a nightmare and was destroying his penis power. He did not compartmentalize. "Don't wait until after supper and the kids have gone to sleep, and you're passing out," I suggested. "Grab your wife and go to bed when you get home, and burn off that stress before it burns you."

A week later he told me he couldn't do it. He thought his wife would feel he was having sex with her only to satisfy his own physical needs and not because he wanted to share the joy of lovemaking with her. This was a noble thought from a man who truly loved his wife, but it was also irrational. I knew his wife, and I urged him to follow my advice despite his reservations. My hunch proved to be correct. His wife thought hopping into bed for a quick, aggressive workout was romantic, and as a result, she was happy to help him burn off stress and not carry it with him all night. A good, loving partner would prefer to see you calm and collected rather than nervous and worried, and if you take care of your partner's needs at the same time you are satisfying your own, you will both end up winners.

Depression Depresses the Penis

Another of the many patients who have come to me thinking they were penis failures was a sweet, gentle man named Bill, an orderly at my hospital. A divorced father of three, Bill developed a bad case of penis weakness after two years of a healthy sex life with his girlfriend. Taking a routine medical history, I found out he had also been sleeping badly and losing weight. When I asked about his state of mind, Bill said he had been depressed. His son was addicted to cocaine and had been caught stealing, and Bill was plagued by feelings of helplessness and remorse. Nothing was wrong with Bill's sexual apparatus. His penis power was on hiatus because of situational depression. Loss of interest in sex is a common and predictable response to deep sadness or personal loss. Instead of letting time take its course, Bill had made the situation worse by forcing himself to have sex with his girlfriend because he feared she would think less of him if he said he did not feel like making love. He went about lovemaking on schedule, but his penis was not ready to perform. In Bill's case, depression was a temporary condition brought on by an identifiable situation. Once he understood the impact of situational depression, he was able to accept that his reaction was normal, and in time, the sadness dissipated. His good life—including his aroused penis—returned.

In other cases, depression can be a chronic, debilitating disease, and its effect on penis power can be long lasting. Such conditions are beyond the scope of a urologist. If you suffer from chronic depression, focusing on your sexuality alone is a mistake. I urge you to see a psychiatrist. Today, medication, psychotherapy, or a combination can effectively manage depression, and with ascent from the depths of depression comes a natural restoration of penis power.

Mind Games

Martin was a middle-aged man who had lost the love of his life a year before he came to see me. After an appropriate period of mourning, he began to say yes when friends set him up with dates. Martin's first few dates were with sexually liberated women. The dates went well, considering that Martin's only sexual experiences outside of marriage had been some furtive encounters with girls when he was very young. But when he finally met a woman he cared for, he suddenly lost his penis power. He could not understand why he performed well with women for whom he felt indifference but not with someone for whom he truly cared.

Martin was plagued by *guilt*, overwhelmed by the thought that as sex with a woman became more intimate and loving, he was betraying his late wife. To spare himself the guilt, his mind "tricked" his penis into falling down on the job. Social norms for relationships, principles of obligation and responsibility, and certain standards or expectations of behavior all contribute to the presence of guilt. Religion is one of the most significant factors. Many of my patients—Christians, Jews, Buddhists, and Muslims—were all perfectly fine sexually within the prescribed context of marriage, but when they indulged in behavior that overstepped the boundaries of their religious precepts, many were driven to penis weakness.

Every person must live by his own morals and ethics. However, anyone who chooses to violate his personal tenets should understand that the subconscious shame can have dramatic effects on the penis, including erectile dysfunction, premature ejaculation, and even a permanent psychological aversion to sex. In most cases, men who struggle with strict religious rules, especially regarding sex, need to talk to a clergyman, not a urologist.

Fears

Another obstacle to penis power is *irrational fear* of a dire consequence when engaging in intercourse. One thirty-year-old man who would have been a virgin had it not been for one woman who coaxed his semierect penis into her vagina came to see me. For this young man, all previous sexual encounters had ended in erection failure or ejaculation before penetration. I referred him to a psychotherapist who discovered that his domineering mother had told him that vaginas had teeth! He never engaged in sexual intercourse because he was plagued by nightmares about getting his member "chewed up."

This patient was an extreme case, but many men fear intercourse for reasons they do not quite understand, and many do not even realize they are afraid. They think they want to have sex. They seek it out, but something always goes wrong, and they conclude that their penises are abnormal. Many of my patients' penises failed them because they feared acquiring some highly unlikely disease like typhoid or were afraid of having a heart attack during sex. These are bizarre terrors rooted in some deeper fear of sex.

Other worries are *not* irrational. Men have good reason to be concerned about sexually transmitted diseases, whether a viral infection such as herpes; a bacterial infection like syphilis, gonorrhea, or chlamydia; or HIV/AIDS. These diseases have been on the increase in recent years. While the others can cause suffering and inhibit your sex life, HIV/AIDS has become the principal sexual scourge in our time because it is incurable and often deadly. The fear of HIV/AIDS has put a definite crimp in the lives of many of my superpotent patients, as well it should, but the time to worry about sexually transmitted diseases is not at the moment of intercourse. You need a game plan long before you get into bed with someone. It is incumbent upon a superpotent man to know a potential sex partner as well as possible before having sex and to have the patience and courage to ask probing questions about that partner's past sexual practices and previous partners. You must make a sound judgment about the truthfulness of your potential partner's answers.

With regard to HIV/AIDS transmission, when you are sexually intimate with any given partner, you are potentially linked to every previous sexual encounter in which your partner has ever indulged. Next time you consider having a one-night stand with a stranger or sleeping with a new partner on a whim, think of the risk. Delaying gratification could end up saving your life.

On the other hand, if *you* are the carrier of any kind of sexually transmitted disease, your absolute duty is to be open and honest with potential partners. If you take sound medical precautions, engage only in safe sexual practices, and exercise sensible sexual judgment, you can be free of fear when it is time to unleash your penis power.

Chapter 8

Extenuating Circumstances: When Sex Becomes a Chore

Larry, a fifty-one-year-old man, came to me for a prostate examination. His prostate was enlarged and would require treatment, possibly even surgery. When I told him, he was relieved. I asked him why he was so happy to hear this. "Because I've been having problems getting it up lately, Doc," he confessed. "I thought maybe I'd become impotent."

"Larry," I said, "I'm sorry to have to tell you this, but if you're having problems with your penis, prostate surgery won't change anything." After all, the prostate's role is to supply seminal fluid to the ejaculate and is unrelated to penis performance.

Larry and I had a long talk, and I learned he had been married to the same woman for nearly thirty years—raising children; dealing with hassles day in and day out; watching each other sag and wrinkle; and having routine, habitual sex. Nothing was wrong with Larry physically. He was suffering from the Coolidge effect.

Researchers studying animal sexuality originally coined the term for a unique behavioral pattern. If you put a male mouse in a cage with a female mouse in heat, he will quickly mount her. After he ejaculates, he will rest before going at it again. This refractory period is predictable. It varies from one species to another but is consistent among all mice, rats, roosters, rams, rhinos, and humans. After the second ejaculation, the refractory period is longer. The same is true after the third, fourth, fifth, and so on. The animal takes longer and longer to recover until it reaches exhaustion.

Here is the interesting part. If at any point you replace the female mouse with a different one, it's back to square one for the male. No matter how many times he has ejaculated, introduce a new female, and his refractory period bounces back to nearly what it might have been after one or two copulations. This is the Coolidge effect.

Why that name? Legend has it that President Calvin Coolidge, the austere conservative they called Silent Cal, once visited a farm with his wife. Noticing an unusually large number of chicks and eggs, Mrs. Coolidge remarked that the few roosters in the barnyard must be prodigious studs. The farmer proudly replied that the roosters did their duty dozens of times a day. "You might point that out to Mr. Coolidge," said the First Lady.

Silent Cal, evidently not as prudish as reputation suggests, asked the farmer if each rooster had to service the same old hen every time. When the farmer said the roosters could mate freely with any hen they wanted, the president responded, "You might point that out to Mrs. Coolidge."

The story may be apocryphal, but it certainly deserves to have an effect named after it.

I have seen Larry's problem in hundreds of men. The situations that cause temporary penis weakness are often so obvious that I am surprised patients don't recognize them. Men are so vulnerable to self-doubt when it comes to penis performance they immediately assume something is wrong with their anatomy when boredom and habituation is to blame. It is true—the thrill of taking off a partner's clothes is not so thrilling when you have unveiled the same body hundreds of times (one survey found that 51 percent of men fantasize about someone else during sex, while only 37 percent of women do).[1] Hearing your partner of twenty-plus years whisper that she wants you is not as exciting as hearing the same words whispered by a shapely stranger. Let's be honest: you do not have to be youth obsessed to be more turned on by a young, lithe body than by the familiar one that gravity and time have altered. Nor do you have to be sexist; I would wager that the same preference holds true for women.

The Hard Dick Syndrome

Nothing will revive a man more quickly and vigorously than a new partner, preferably someone young, attractive, and receptive. While that observation may seem subversive to those who cherish the spiritual and emotional benefits of lasting love, when it comes to penis power, the evidence speaks loud and clear. Men who have difficulty making love to their longtime partners can be dynamos with their secret lovers. Men can be troubled by penis problems until they get separated or divorced and suddenly find rejuvenation with a new lover.

It is not my place to endorse any particular lifestyle, but penis weakness is often circumstantial, and the Coolidge effect defines one of the primary circumstances. That said, men who assume new is always better should realize that such thinking can be dangerous. I have seen too many men jeopardize, and sometimes forfeit, longstanding relationships of immense value because they followed their penises in pursuit of a newer, younger partner.

Many men solve their boredom problems *temporarily*, only to realize later that they desperately miss the love and companionship they squandered. Their penises are reborn for a little while, only to retreat again when the new love grows stale. *Beware of the hard dick syndrome!* After a while, it can turn into the Coolidge effect.

Solutions to the Coolidge effect can often be found within the confines of a good, monogamous relationship. Those same animal researchers found that the male's vigor can return, even without a new female, if something else is altered—a new scent, a new look on a familiar mate (the researchers achieved this by painting the female mouse's coat a new color). The lesson here for humans, both male and female, is that familiarity might not breed contempt, but it does breed boredom. Break old, tired habits. Change your routines. Use your imagination. Make love in different places or at different times. Wear different clothing. Daub yourself with unusual scents. Try different positions. Whatever it takes to bring a sense of adventure to your sex life, do it! Do not give up on yourself by thinking you have suddenly become impotent.

Problems that stem from longevity and familiarity might seem contradictory to the notion that fear and performance anxiety can cause penis failure during first encounters. You may wonder if I am suggesting that being with an exciting new partner for the first time can cause temporary penis failure the same way that penis failure can be caused by being with the same partner for a long period of time. The answer is yes, another Penis Paradox.

Both sets of circumstances can cause the same types of problems for very different reasons. First-time problems result because the situation is *too* exciting, and anticipation of sex, apprehension, and anxiety over your performance may become heightened, causing you to lose an erection or ejaculate too quickly.

With a longtime partner, the problem arises not because of first-time jitters but because of diminished desire and a need for more time and more direct stimulation to get aroused. If you do not add some imagination to the routine, you might find your penis lying down on the job.

The solution to the first-time anxiety is to cultivate a comfortable, relaxed, familiar relationship. If *that* reaches a critical mass and the problem of monotony sets in, the antidote is to generate excitement with freshness and variety.

One fifty-five-year-old patient who was married to a woman he loved for twenty-seven years had a bad case of sexual ennui that led to a brief fling. At home he was now inhibited by guilt and boredom. "Jack," I said, "take Friday off; get your wife to cancel all her plans. Rent a cabin in the mountains. Tune out the world. No kids, no phone, no television—just the two of you and a fireplace."

The weekend rejuvenated Jack and his wife, as similar escapes have done for countless couples. In other cases, I have advised patients to surprise their wives with flowers and a sunset tryst in a motel. Other couples pretend they have just met and are having a one-night stand.

Others vary their rituals. If you have been initiating sex after you are both washed, undressed, and in bed, try doing it before all of those bedtime rituals. When was the last time you and your partner undressed each other or necked in the living room or made love in the kitchen or shower? Have you tried a different position? Used props? Browse in any sex shop, and you'll find countless ideas for invigorating your sex life. Some of my patients have to be told that sex is not just a nighttime activity. Why engage in something as important as sex when your body is at its lowest energy level? Perhaps your penis problem is really a fatigue problem. The penis, like hormonal secretions and energy levels, responds to different biorhythms. Concrete scientific evidence to validate this observation is sparse at this time, but research is ongoing.

Fatigue affects sexual energy, and so I encourage my patients to pay close attention to the ways in which their bodies, and especially their penises, respond to different emotional and physical conditions. Being aware that your sexual responsiveness will change with stress, fatigue, anxiety, or sickness is fundamentally important. Your body's rhythms may be better suited to sex at unusual times of the day. Exercise, diet, or work schedules may affect your sex drive. Don't feel burdened by sex. Take the initiative to spice things up, and you won't be disappointed.

Hard on Demand

Millions of men think that something is wrong with them because they do not get "hard on demand." Our culture's pervasive myth has it that a real man will be raring to go anytime, day or night. The truth is each man has his own individual preferences and unique biological templates. There is no set time or place you are supposed to get aroused. No credible scientific book says you have to have sex a certain number of times a day to be a real man. Some men tell me they feel sexiest in the morning, some in the middle of the night. The real problem is that most men are too inhibited to break old habits or are afraid their partners will think they are crazy for trying something new. If you are passionate and exciting, your partner most likely will not complain.

Morning sex is an especially good way to break the routine. So what if you have to skip jogging, rush through breakfast, or reach work a bit late? Morning sex clears the spirit of any tension and shakes the cobwebs out of your body. A lot of men like sex better in the morning because they wake up with the so-called morning wood, caused by a full bladder compressing the venous outflow from the pelvic vessels, which then hold blood in the penis longer than usual. Be assured that after morning lovemaking, you will like what you see in the mirror.

If you are a man who wants to enhance your penis power, or if you are a partner who wants to learn how to increase your man's penis power, it behooves you to look into alternative sex practices. The possibilities are endless. If you cannot conjure up some creative ideas on your own, do not be afraid to go out and find a book or ask a friend for tips. Any change should add a fresh dimension to your routine.

Be Careful!

I must add an important caveat: *draw the line at unprotected anal intercourse*. This practice is highly risky, even with the use of a condom. In the last twenty-five years, people who practice anal sex, or are tempted to, have become increasingly concerned about HIV/AIDS. This concern is justified. Thinking of anal intercourse as an occasional treat is not safe. All studies indicate that a primary mode of transmission of HIV/AIDS is through anal sex. The anus is particularly vulnerable to tears in the delicate tissue membrane, which expose the perianal blood vessels as a port of entry for the deadly retrovirus. Unprotected anal sex should be off limits on the basis of the HIV/AIDS risk alone, and couples indulging in such practices should be aware that anal sex brings other health risks as well. If the penis enters the rectum and comes in contact with fecal matter (which contains toxic bacteria, particularly E. coli), this can cause major infections in the prostate, bladder, kidneys, or blood. If the infection spreads to the bloodstream, it can result in sepsis, a potentially fatal infection that causes the body's immune system to attack its own organs and tissues. In addition, if the penis is inserted into the rectum and then inserted into the vagina, it can contaminate the nearby urethra with fecal matter and cause a severe bladder infection in a female partner.

"Blow" Is Not an Accurate Description

Oral sex is another story entirely. The act itself has made many a reluctant penis as hard as a diamond. The sucking action creates a vacuum effect that transmits a negative filling pressure to the blood vessels within the penile shaft, drawing blood into its channels. Psychologically, oral sex can also add excitement. What a thrill for a man to experience his partner doing something so loving and gracious. Many of my older patients have told me that the sucking action of oral sex is the *only* way they can obtain an erection firm enough for penetration, all the more reason to use oral sex as a way to improve your sex life.

Many women have a negative attitude toward oral sex. Some feel that it puts them in a subservient position, while some find it physically unpleasant if the man's penis touches the pharynx in the back of the throat. This can initiate the gag reflex. Some women complain that oral sex is a one-way street. All these concerns are legitimate and understandable, but the fact is there are many ways to position your body for oral sex—you do not have to be on your knees. A woman can also ask the man to refrain from thrusting his pelvis during oral sex to avoid the gag reflex. All good sexual relationships entail giving and receiving. If a woman performs oral sex for her man, there is no harm in asking for something special in return, and most women I meet in my practice *enjoy* giving and receiving oral sex. They find the act erotic, and many say it gives them a greater degree of control than other types of foreplay.

If your partner is reluctant to perform oral sex, explain the physiology—why it gets a rise out of a penis. Allow your partner to express the reasons for her reservations. Try to assure your partner that oral sex is not inherently dangerous (although partners should be aware of each other's past sexual experiences), dirty, or sinful. If your partner had a bad experience, assure her that you care for her too much to hurt her in any way, and let her know that her trying again would mean a lot to you. It just might add a whole new dimension to your sex lives.

A Time and Place for Everything

Gary was a young engineer who married his college sweetheart right after college graduation. Soon after, they had a child. The marriage was going well, but that changed when the company Gary worked for was hurt by a recession and Gary was laid off. When he told me he was having penis problems, I assumed it was because his self-esteem had taken a blow as a result of the layoff. This is common. When a man suffers a financial setback or comes up short in his career goals, his masculinity takes a beating, and this can manifest in penis failure, as if the mind says, "You messed up your career; you are less of a man, so you must also be inadequate sexually."

Understanding the importance of this link between the health of your penis power and your ability to achieve success in other endeavors is essential. Gary had enough insight to realize that the layoff was an unfortunate turn of events that, in reality, had no bearing on his masculinity, and at first, his sex life was not diminished. When his job hunting turned up nothing and the financial pressure mounted, he was forced to move his family into his parents' home, a temporary remedy during which he found his penis power dropping like the profits of his former company.

The reason? He was sleeping in the bedroom he used for eighteen years, the bedroom in which he self-consciously masturbated, hoping his parents, whose room was nearby, would not barge in. This was the bedroom where he sneaked dates and nervously tried to have sex before his parents got home. Just being in that room triggered all the sexual anxieties of his adolescence. The worries were subconscious but the anxiety was perfectly obvious to his penis. When I suggested that the house might be the problem, Gary tested the hypothesis by checking into a motel with his wife. They had a sizzling weekend. As a result, he was able to laugh at the whole episode and quickly made different living arrangements.

Gary's situation is unusual, but it illustrates the relationship between *environment* and penis power. Location may not be as important in sex as it is in real estate, but it can play a major role in your ability to perform adequately. Noise, the wrong temperature, the possibility of being interrupted, lighting, and negative associations can affect your penis performance. True, a superpotent man should rise to the challenge regardless of his environment, but everyone has preferences. Some men like hard-driving rock 'n' roll while they romp with their lovers; some prefer violins. Some men like the room totally dark; some like candlelight. Some men are inhibited by the proximity of others, and some find the danger of discovery a turnon.

What mood, setting, or location puts you in a sexual state of mind? Arrange your sexual trysts to suit those preferences, or at least avoid situations that diminish your penis power. If you are not sure of your preferences, don't be afraid to experiment until you find just what you are looking for.

The Sweet Smell of Success

Carl was a twenty-five-year-old actor with an enviable history of superpotent adventures. One day he fell madly in love. The sex was fantastic and so was the emotional connection. After a whirlwind few weeks, the couple moved in together. Shortly thereafter, Carl started having erection failures. I was sure I knew what the problem was. I had seen it before. "Carl," I said, "living with someone for the first time is terrifying. You feel trapped, my boy, afraid of losing your freedom. Fear is expressing itself through your penis."

Carl said he was happy to be living with someone. He felt he was even *more* free because he had someone he loved to come home to. So I probed. Had anything changed since she moved in?

They had not had a fight. She had not issued ultimatums. She had not stopped wanting sex. Then he told me that the odor from her vagina had become unpleasant to him. When they were dating, she was conscientious about her hygiene, but now she didn't always have the time or motivation to tend to herself.

A macho guy, Carl thought nothing as trivial as an odor should interfere with his penis power, so he blamed himself. Still, he found his girlfriend's scent so distasteful that no matter how aroused he was he became *unaroused* the moment she removed her panties, but he did not have the heart to tell her.

Having examined thousands of women in my practice, I have adopted the attitude of an environmental engineer when it comes to hygiene. The vagina presents a number of unique conditions. Anatomically, it is a deep cavity with a relatively small opening and a large potential for expandable space within. It houses a variety of natural secretions and gets little ventilation or light. This makes it a breeding ground for bacteria and yeast. It takes some modest effort for some women to keep their vaginas clean and pleasant smelling, and many women do not realize the effect that a strong, unpleasant scent can have on a man.

All women should make vaginal hygiene a priority, for their general health and also so that an odor does not interfere with romantic relationships. The same adherence to maintaining hygiene applies to men, who have just as much potential to emit bad odors from their penises.

I told Carl it was vital to *communicate* exactly how he felt. With two adults in a good relationship, one partner should be able to suggest they both wash before getting intimate. Taking a shower together before sex is a great way to steam things up. Odors might not be a romantic topic, but it is the second most unpleasant aspect of sex and deserves to be discussed openly.

The Most Unpleasant Aspect of Sex

I know what you're thinking: If odor is in second place, what's in first? Sixty percent of the men whom I surveyed answered "an unresponsive partner."

What makes a penis the hardest is an *enthusiastic lover* in an equally conducive environment. This is due to both the psychological lift a man gets from knowing that he is capable of exciting a desirable partner and the physiological response men have to stimulating their partner. The penis responds to warmth, moisture, erotic sounds, tight embraces, and any other sign of satisfaction.

The opposite is also true. Too many men take it personally when a lover fails to respond, automatically assuming something is wrong with *them*. The worst scenario is when a man, out of panic and fear, does not respond to the unresponsive partner. This nonresponse usually leads to a destructive chain of *nonreactions*, and ultimately men think their penises have failed them. This is ridiculous. At some point in every man's sexual lifespan, he will have to deal with an unresponsive lover.

It is important to be sensitive to the delicate clues your partner gives you and to communicate in an open, honest, considerate way. Talk to your partner about her mood, and try to get her mind off distractions. If there is a conflict within the relationship, work it out before continuing to have sex. If you find yourself with an unresponsive partner, move slowly and explore the sensuality of the experience, paying close attention to the subtle body language of your lover. Be persistent and diligent, delicate and precise. Learn everything you can about your partner's sexuality and preferences. What turns her on? If necessary, make an effort to expand your sexual repertoire and learn some new tricks. More importantly, do not blame yourself for what you cannot control. Ultimately, if you pay attention to the delicate cues of an unresponsive partner and use every weapon in your sexual arsenal, you can make what was once a difficult situation a delight.

If you have tried your best, and your partner is still unresponsive, forgive yourself and move on. Your partner might have a serious hangup that is beyond your ability to fix, or you might be sexually incompatible. It happens. Unfortunately, sometimes incompatibility develops *after* a couple has been having satisfying sex. If that happens and you want the relationship to continue, by all means avail yourselves of counseling or therapy. Do *something* before it becomes disastrous to your emotional and sexual well-being.

It pains me to say that many of my patients are stuck with partners who do nothing to satisfy a man's desires, and those men too often blame themselves and sometimes run to their urologist for help. They do not need a urologist. They need to figure out how to remedy their situation or move on before their penises die a premature death.

Intimate Intimidation

There is an old joke that goes like this: There are two gates into heaven. Above one gate is a sign that reads, "Men Who Are Intimidated by Women." An endless line stretches out from this gate. Above the other gate is this sign: "Men Who Are Not Intimidated by Women." Only one highly unattractive guy stands in line at this gate.

Intrigued, Saint Peter walks up to him and says, "Tell me, my son, what qualifies you to be in this line?"

The man replies, "My wife told me to stand here."

Every man, even the strongest, most self-assured, and independent superpotent man, at some time or another has felt intimidated by a woman. That is one of the deep secrets men carry. The strong ones laugh about it; the weak ones deny it. One fact is undeniable: a relentlessly intimidating partner is anathema to penis power.

What do I mean by intimidating? Most men like sexually aggressive partners who let them know what they want and are up-front about their desires. Every man has his own line that separates the kind of aggressiveness that arouses him from the kind that makes him want to run away. When aggressiveness is perceived as demanding or threatening, it can cause penis problems.

Aggressive and demanding lovers put pressure on men to perform incredible feats of sexual wonder (at least that is what intimidated men think). An overtly challenging demand can sound like a military command, "Get hard now!" That is tough for any man, especially if the intimidator is really saying, "I don't think you are man enough for me. And if you're not, I'm going to let you know about it." Even if you have no previous history of penis weakness, a new set of overly aggressive demands can trigger the self-doubt that lurks deep within the male psyche: *Can* I satisfy you? Will I measure up? What if I don't? And once you start thinking those negative thoughts, you'll have penis failure.

If you are with someone who has unrealistic expectations or puts too much pressure on you to perform, communicate your feelings. Tell him how it makes you feel when he sets up unrealistic standards. If communication does not change his attitude, you may have to consider the possibility that he is not suitable as a partner for you. Do not be fooled into thinking that a real man should meet crazy demands without blinking or that failing to do so is a sign of personal inadequacy.

Many caring, good-hearted lovers intimidate men without even realizing it. One of my patients had been with his new girlfriend for six months, and everything was going well. One night they ran into her ex-boyfriend who looked like a movie star and had the body of an all-pro halfback. My patient's girlfriend later told him the ex-boyfriend was sexually unstoppable. "He could go all night."

Her intention was innocent. The heart of her story was that the ex-boyfriend's abusiveness was obscured by his sexual prowess, and that had been an important lesson for her. She thought she was sharing openly, but her words had a chilling effect. My patient started wondering how his sexual performance compared to her ex-boyfriend's. He grew fearful that he would lose her by not matching up. The result was an outbreak of penis weakness. After he and I spoke, he told her and learned that his fear was all in his head. The girlfriend adored him and was not comparing him sexually to the other man (at least she was smart enough to *say* she was not).

Whether real or imaginary, deliberate or unintentional, never compare your performance to some hypothetical standard. Give each sexual encounter your best effort, and you'll feel good about yourself. Live with your penis and cherish it for what it is. It does not matter if there are, or were, other men out there who can outperform you. If I were to compare myself to Tiger Woods every time I play golf, I would never tee off again. Just be yourself, and never stop striving to become the best lover you can be.

When the Problem Is in Your Heart

Marty was a forty-seven-year-old business agent in terrific physical shape and had acquired a reputation as a superpotent bachelor before he married Marilyn. He told me after two years of marriage, "I don't feel like making love to my wife lately, and when I do, I'm not the man I used to be. Check my testosterone level."

I did the blood test to satisfy him, but I already knew Marty's testosterone was normal. The previous weekend, I had seen Marty and his wife arguing heatedly in public. In the office I asked him how their relationship was. His answer was circumspect. I could tell from his body language that he was harboring anger.

"Go straighten things out between you and Marilyn, and your penis will straighten out, too." I charged him an extra thirty-five cents for the psychiatric consultation.

From my clinical experience, I long ago concluded that the greatest aphrodisiac ever invented is love itself. The opposite is also true: *the biggest enemy of sexual desire is hate*. Nothing will make a penis slink away and hide as quickly as anger, hostility, or resentment toward a partner. If a man fails to express his feelings, the situation gets worse. When he goes through the motions of making love, his penis says, "I'm not getting hard for that!"

If you are harboring animosity toward your partner, if you are rehashing angry feelings in your head without expressing them, if resentment has been accumulating in your heart so much that it obscures the love that brought you together, how can it not affect what happens in bed?

With long-term partners especially, the heart rules the penis. As time goes by, the fires of passion diminish, and more than anything else, the emotions guide the course of sexuality. It is beyond the scope of this book and my professional expertise to advise you on all the complexities of romantic and sexual relationships and the nuances of subtle emotions. What I can do is tell you what I tell my patients: *remove anger and resentment from your relationship, and your love life will be strong and long lasting.*

Do not take your partner for granted. Do not let your appreciation wane. Do not let petty animosities overshadow the qualities that have kept you together. Two mature people with a strong commitment have the greatest potential for mutually satisfying sex. This does not mean that problems will not arise. Every relationship has conflicts, and you must be aware that every conflict affects your penis. You also have to be aware that the most effective response to a conflict is to work through the problems in a healthy and effective way. Communicate. If you cannot do it on your own, find a counselor or a friend who can help you to get your feelings out in the open. That does not just mean venting.

It means truly discussing the issues in an atmosphere of fairness and mutual respect.

Chapter 9

As Old as You Feel: The Life Story of the Penis

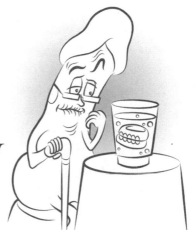

I s it not strange that desire should so many years outlive per-formance?" Shakespeare eloquently and perceptively noted.[1] It might seem strange to men whose penis power appears to diminish with age, but it is certainly not strange to a urologist. Of all the circumstances that affect the functioning of a penis, the most predictable is the normal, inevitable process of aging.

By far, the most frequent complaint I hear is a variation on the following: "Something's wrong, Doc. I am not the man I used to be." What men usually mean is that they do not have the same level of *sexual desire* they once had; that it takes longer to get an erection, longer to ejaculate, longer to get aroused again after they make love; that their erections are not as firm; or some or all of the above. All are predictable changes that occur as men get older. They happen at different times to different men, but they happen to every man who lives long enough.

Problems arise with either of two responses to the aging process: (1) the patient does not realize that such changes are normal and concludes that he has a medical or psychological problem, or (2) he *does* know that these developments are typical and concludes that he is hopelessly over the hill. Both conclusions are wrong.

A typical example of the first kind of man is a radiologist colleague who was approaching his fiftieth birthday. He was a man of superpotency and excellent general fitness. Noticing cramps in his legs while running, he saw an internist and was diagnosed with claudication, a condition characterized by cramping of the leg muscles while exercising. This is caused by diminished blood flow, usually the result of arteriosclerotic plaque blocking the arteries supplying blood to the legs.

The radiologist concluded that if the blood flow in his legs had become impeded, the same might also be true of the blood supply to his penis. My colleague had been alarmed for some time by the decline in his penis power, and this was the explanation he had been searching for. His ego had prevented him from saying anything to me, but now that he was sure it was a medical problem, he came to me for treatment. After a complete uro-vascular profile, I was able to say without reservation that the blood flow to his penis was nearly as good as it had been when he was thirty. I suggested a little help from vasoactive pills. His penis power was still high, but his erections were not as firm as they used to be. "Do you run as far as you did at twenty-five?" I asked him. "Can you lift as much weight? Dance until dawn?" No one expects that, nor should you expect your penis to be as firm at age fifty as it was at age twenty.

The second kind of man is the one who is worn out, ailing, cynical, and prone to complaining about life in general. He may interpret changes in his sexuality as a sign of impending death and put his penis out to pasture without even a gold watch or a ceremony.

The key point to remember is that as you age, you do not lose penis power, and your penis performance does not become inferior. It simply changes. Unless you have a legitimate medical disorder that interferes with your penis functioning, you can be as superpotent at eighty as you were at twenty.

Penis Passages

From birth until puberty, the penis is basically a conduit for urine, but the mechanism of erection is present even before birth. All male children, including infants, get erections. These are involuntary and occur due to nerve stimulation. They can be caused by a full bladder or by rubbing the penis with a towel after bathing. They are not associated with anything sexual.

Then comes puberty. The testicles have developed to the point where they produce enough circulating testosterone to alter the size and appearance of certain body parts. At this stage, a boy develops *secondary sexual characteristics*, including facial, underarm, and pubic hair; a deeper voice; adult-size genitalia; and the ability to ejaculate. Suddenly, the penis is a wonderful novelty! Adolescents cannot play with theirs enough. Simply looking at a sexy picture or a girl's legs can stimulate the young penis to a full erection. Teens realize they can masturbate and inevitably discover that it can be even nicer with a partner.

Typically, in their late teens, boys become sexually obsessed. The level of desire, the ease with which they become aroused, and their capacity for frequent sex are astounding. Dominated by hormones, physically fit, and not yet burdened by adult responsibilities, the teenage male is a walking erection, capable of getting one at any time with little or no provocation and ejaculating five or six times a day! At no time does the penis rule the brain more than it does in adolescence.

A professor of mine at Princeton once brought down the house with a cogent observation about young men in college. Princeton was not yet coed when I was an undergraduate. The auditorium was filled with a few hundred male freshmen in a philosophy survey course. Our professor looked us over and said, "If there were any way to channel the mental energy you all have focused on your collective dicks into a more productive intellectual plane, I might find a Nobel laureate out there, and surely most of you would go through college Phi Beta Kappa and summa cum laude while saving a hell of a lot of energy!"

The Early Years

The penis problems I treat in patients in their late teens and early twenties are typically those associated with hypersensitivity. The young man who is nervous about whether he is as normal or as virile as his friends might lose his perpetual erection at precisely the wrong moment. More typical is the problem of premature ejaculation. As discussed in chapter 3, the adolescent penis is extremely sensitive, the volume of semen produced is higher than at any other stage of life, and the young man usually has not had enough experience to develop self-control. He might ejaculate before penetration or immediately thereafter. If only he knew how typical this was!

The solution for most young men is simply to have more frequent ejaculations. (A cautionary note: frequent sex should not be regarded as synonymous with indiscriminate sex.) For men in their late teens and early twenties, the refractory period can be as short as a few minutes. If you ejaculated prematurely the first time, the next time you will last longer because less fluid is in your seminal vesicles and you have less physiological urgency to release it. A higher level of stimulation over a longer period of time is required to get through the excitatory phase to when the reflex of ejaculation occurs.

Penis weakness for men in their early to late twenties almost never stems from something physical though, medically speaking, the peak of sexuality might have been passed at nineteen or twenty. The young men in this group are usually out of school and suddenly making grown-up decisions. The big man on campus is now the little man in the office. The coeds he picked up in classrooms and fraternity houses are now young women with whom he might be in a real relationship. For the first time, he is working long, hard hours. All of this often leads to a high level of *stress*, and most young men have not yet developed the ability to *compartmentalize*. Self-doubt can occur and lead to unwanted penis consequences.

Is It Ageless?

From the peak period of sexuality until your penis is laid to rest with your other organs at life's end, other changes occur that will not be seen in the penis itself. This is another Penis Paradox: agelessness. While your other organs degenerate—skin wrinkles, waistline expands, hair grays and vanishes—your aging penis undergoes virtually no change in size or appearance as you age. The trained eye of a urologist might discern a subtle difference between a twenty-year-old and an eighty-year-old penis; the elderly penis has relaxed suspensory ligaments (located just under the pubic bone), giving the impression that the penis has lengthened. This is illusory. The penis is not longer; it is just drooping. Conversely, there is no *shrinkage* of the penis with age.

What does change with age is how the penis behaves. Older men first notice that it takes longer to get an erection. This begins to happen to men in their twenties, but so gradually that most men don't notice until they approach middle age. Much depends on the kinds of relationships they have and the frequency of sexual activity. Once your testosterone levels diminish with age, fantasies are no longer enough; the mere sight of a sexy body or heated foreplay might not do it. Many older men can only get an erection from the vacuum effect of oral sex and the psychological aspects associated with that sexual act. You might also notice that sometimes your erections as you age are only half-hard or semi-rigid until added stimulation hopefully brings them to full strength. This, too, is normal, but men often panic, recalling the days when they spent half their time concealing their erections.

The same is true of the refractory period. The amount of time it takes to recover after an ejaculation increases and the volume of the ejaculate decreases in proportion to a man's age. When a man reaches his fifties and sixties, the refractory period might be as long as twenty-four hours, even with direct stimulation. At eighty, it might be one week. Men also notice that the ejaculation itself feels less and less explosive as they age; the semen leaks out rather than being forcefully expelled. Orgasms might feel less intense. All this is a normal part of the aging process. The good news is that with age comes increased experience, wisdom, and seasoning, which should be a boon to your sex life. An old story illustrates this fact. An old bull and a young bull are roaming the plains of Wyoming when they come upon a ridge overlooking a valley filled with thirty grazing cows. The young bull jumps excitedly up and down, shouting, "Let's *run* down this hill as fast as we can and screw us a few cows!" The old bull, surveying the situation, turns ever so calmly to his young companion and says, "Son, how about we mosey on down there *real slow* and screw them *all!*"

The point is that as you age, your body may not be as flexible, your sex drive may diminish, and your erections may not be as firm, but you can use your wisdom and sexual insight to your advantage. You and your partner can enjoy the extra foreplay required to get you ready. Focus your attention on getting the absolute most out of the intercourse you can handle. Do not be let down if your ejaculations are not as volcanic as they once were—you can still enjoy the pleasure of orgasm well into old age.

As you age, not only do you naturally acquire greater ejaculatory control, but also you should have learned a great deal about pleasing a partner in general, and your partner in particular. You should have learned tricks for arousing and satisfying the person with whom you share your bed.

As you reach your sixties and seventies, you may have to adjust your *style* of lovemaking. Your penis might look as young as ever, but the rest of you has aged. You might have more control over when you ejaculate, but your arms might not be strong enough to support you for as long as they used to do. The muscles in your back and legs might tire quickly, and your joints and ligaments might not be as flexible. This may mean you have to rest or change positions more often. You might have to try different positions. And you'll want to maintain a healthy lifestyle, making it a priority to have a healthy diet and a vigorous exercise regimen.

Another change should be viewed as a bonus: it takes *longer* to reach orgasm. As the old joke goes, "It takes all night to do what I used to do all night long," but this is not a problem, especially if you found it difficult to control your ejaculations in the past. Also, if your partner is a woman, she may even get more pleasure because bringing a woman to

orgasm is usually easier with prolonged intercourse, and the more satisfied your partner is, the more aroused *you* will be.

Some men take *too* long to ejaculate in general, not just as they age,
a problem usually associated with a reduced level of sensitivity in the
penis or a habitual mind-set that views prolonged sex as the only way
to achieve orgasm, or both. Because some partners may find prolonged
sex irritating, painful, or unpleasant, I recommend prolonging foreplay, trying new positions, and otherwise addressing whatever issues
may be causing the problem. Men must make the appropriate adjustments to accommodate their partners' comfort level. Communication,
awareness, and consideration are the best triad to navigate the intricate
workings of a sexual relationship.

When the Going Gets Tough: Male Menopause and TRT

Similar to what happens to women during menopause, for men over
forty, testosterone levels start to fall at an average of about 1 percent
per year. As indestructible teenagers, testosterone helped build our
muscles and develop strong bones. As young men, record-setting levels
of testosterone made us heroes on the gridiron, boosted our energy,
and propelled our foolish actions with the false belief that our youthful
bodies could scale an unattainable mountaintop.

As urologists learn more about the role of testosterone in the physical and mental development of young men in their prime, we are also
studying the role of testosterone in the aging body. Testosterone replacement therapy (TRT) has been promoted in the print media and
television and especially over the Internet as the solution to the male
equivalent of menopause (andropause). TRT promises improvement
to a man's libido, increased muscle mass, elimination of cognitive defi-
ciencies, elevation of mood, and a bolster to bone density.

Progressive testosterone (androgen) deficiency in aging men has led
to a syndrome known as hypogonadism, which can manifest in osteopo-
rosis (loss of bone density), decreased libido, erectile dysfunction, and
mood changes ("grumpy old man syndrome"). In addition, hypogonadism causes muscles to become flabby and decrease in size, leaving men

with middle-age paunch. As hypogonadism has become more widely recognized, physicians have enormously increased the number of testosterone replacement prescriptions. Pharmaceutical statistics indicate a 500 percent increase in the use of testosterone products in the elderly and middle-aged population.[2]

Who Needs Testosterone Replacement?

For a physician to determine if a patient needs TRT, blood levels of testosterone must be assessed. The accepted low limit for normal adult men is a testosterone level of at least 200 ng/dl (nanograms per deciliter). If a man's serum testosterone is below 200 ng/dl, TRT is recommended. If a man's serum testosterone level falls between 200 and 400 ng/dl, it is a gray zone as the risk-to-benefit ratio and attendant hazards must be considered. All potential risks of TRT must be discussed between the patient and his doctor. For serum testosterone levels of greater than 400 ng/dl, not only is there *no benefit* to TRT, but also there is considerable risk involved. Men who are experiencing some of the symptoms of andropause should consult a physician, have their serum testosterone checked, and determine how best to proceed with treatment, if any.

The Risks of TRT: Good News, but at a Price

For me, the main areas of concern for long-term effects of TRT are cardiovascular and prostate problems, both of which are commonly found in men with diminished testosterone levels. Cardiologists note that the increased incidence of coronary artery disease in men, compared with women, may be testosterone dependent. Men receiving long-term TRT have been found to have significant changes in their lipid profiles that directly affect cardiovascular health. The bad news is that TRT lowers the beneficial cholesterol (high density lipids, or HDL) widely recognized for its role in protecting against coronary artery disease. The good news is that TRT *also* lowers the bad cholesterol (low density lipids, or LDL) responsible for blocking coronary arteries. These effects on the lipid profile may be minimal when TRT maintains a serum testosterone level below 400 ng/dl. But the cardiac risks increase dramatically when TRT is taken to abusive or supraphysiological levels above 500 ng/dl.

TRT also results in increased production of red blood cells causing a hypercoagulation of the blood, a thickening that may increase the potential for a stroke or heart attack. This is especially true in smokers, who already have an increased circulating red blood cell volume. I do not recommend TRT that raises serum testosterone above 400 ng/dl. Having a healthy heart and healthy arteries should not be compromised by the desire for a slender waistline or bodybuilder muscles.

If you start TRT, do not exceed the recommended dosage in an attempt to radically change your physical appearance. To the aging man who longs for that youthful body, my advice is to modify your diet, maintain a healthy exercise routine, and accept the reality of aging that sometimes brings with it a little paunch.

In addition, it is well known that TRT *does not* induce the development of prostate cancer; however, it can cause rapid and potentially catastrophic growth of an unrecognized prostate cancer. Even with a tiny focus of cancerous cells in an otherwise benign prostate, TRT can encourage these cells to grow explosively and potentially become life threatening. In my clinical experience, the incidence of prostate cancer in patients who have been on TRT for at least six months is no more than the rate of prostate cancer among men not taking testosterone. But if a man is receiving TRT, his doctor should meticulously monitor his prostate health with a periodic digital rectal examination (DRE), cancer screening blood tests (PSA test), and prostatic ultrasonography.

In my judgment, using TRT is safe and clearly beneficial in *symptomatic* men with a serum testosterone level of less than 200 ng/dl. In men whose serum testosterone is greater than 400 ng/dl, it is *unacceptable*.

Unfortunately, all oral preparations of testosterone have been abandoned in the United States because of severe liver toxicity. An acceptable alternative is intramuscular injection. This is relatively inexpensive but dosing is intermittent, which means that the highest levels of serum testosterone are achieved shortly after the injection. Toward the end of the cycle, which usually lasts two to three weeks, the blood level of serum testosterone has diminished to pretreatment levels, and the effect of the circulating testosterone is variable. Implantable testosterone pellets are also available and have the advantage of producing a more stable level of serum testosterone, but this treatment modality is expensive and cumbersome.

Over the past several years, an exciting new treatment modality for TRT known as transdermal application has been developed. Transdermal preparations allow the testosterone to be applied directly to the skin with a patch or a gel, and absorption occurs through the skin and into the bloodstream, resulting in a normal, steady, and effective level of circulating serum testosterone over a twenty-four-hour period. The transdermal patches often cause skin irritation, known as contact dermatitis; more desirable is the transdermal gel, either Testim 1 percent or AndroGel, applied on a non-hair-bearing surface. Testosterone gels are relatively expensive when compared to the cost per month for injectable testosterone. Your best choice is to find a treatment modality that suits both your physical and financial needs.

Young at Heart, Young in Person

I cannot reiterate this point enough: *attitude* is the key to penis longevity. My superpotent patients tell me that sex gives them as much joy at seventy as it did at twenty, and some say it is even better! Many of my older patients, even those who are wealthy, choose not to retire; they cut back their hours and delegate responsibility to others, but they remain active, both in work and in play. These individuals tend to be my healthiest, most superpotent patients. They live longer, and the quality of their lives seems better than those who retire.

Until recently, our society's image of aging usually excluded sex. I know elderly people who have to sneak around to have sex just as they did when they were teenagers because they know their peers and children will frown on it. The generation I now see entering their senior years are recognizing that they deserve active, healthy sex lives as long as they remain physically fit. It will not harm them unless they try positions their muscles and joints are too weak to manage, or they overextend themselves to the point of exhaustion.

Adjust your sexual activities as your body changes, and look upon the adjustment as both a new challenge and a new opportunity. As you age, learn to use your imagination to make up in creativity what you may lack in physical strength. You can stay superpotent as you age by maintaining good overall health habits: exercising regularly; minimizing your consumption of fat and cholesterol; controlling your weight; refraining from smoking, excessive drinking, and drugs; watching your blood pressure; and seeing your physician regularly.

Most importantly, *do not think old*! Your body may produce less testosterone, your blood vessels may become partially obstructed and diminish blood flow to the penis, and your muscles and joints may begin to deteriorate. But if your mind is strong, your penis can be strong, too. Think of yourself as a singer whose voice is not as powerful as it once was, but who more than makes up for it with phrasing, feeling, and subtlety or as an athlete or dancer whose legs are no longer as strong as oaks but who performs with added grace shaped by the wisdom of experience. If you keep your enthusiasm, you can compensate for, or even delay, the effects of aging.

The strenuous use of your penis will sharpen your mind, exalt your soul, and keep you feeling vigorous. In short, you do not stop having sex because you get old, *you get old because you stop having sex*!

The golden years often mean you do not have to get up and go to the office in the morning or worry as much about kids and bills; you have less daily stress and fewer pressures, and you have more privacy, more time, and the luxury of patience. This is an opportunity for a superpotent man to make the most of his penis power.

Andropause versus Menopause

We should acknowledge that as long-term couples age, significant changes occur in both partners. For the most part, postmenopausal women have a *decreased* sex drive, due largely to the marked decrease in estrogen (analogous to testosterone) that accompanies menopause, as well as the psychological effects of an aging body. Many women become depressed during menopause, and a caring partner must be sensitive, using compassion and patience both inside and outside of the bedroom.

In many aging women, as estrogen levels start to fall, it becomes increasingly difficult for the vagina to lubricate itself. Topical estrogen and a variety of lubricants can be used effectively and safely. Postmenopausal women have a far greater *disinterest* in sex than do men experiencing andropause. For this reason, the superpotent man must adjust his expectations and talk candidly to his partner about these changes. Above all, do not turn your back on your lifelong partner for a younger, more responsive lover. A young, sexy lover might make you feel like a stud, but very quickly you'll find that sacrificing the friendship, intimacy, and bond of a long-term relationship might not be worth the quick fix.

Sex is not only safe for older couples, it is also good for them, maintaining overall physical strength and cardiovascular health and keeping them invigorated.

Penis Posterity

Even if aging has reduced your body's capacity, medical science is capable of helping you maintain your penis power. We know the single most common cause of erectile dysfunction with aging is arteriosclerosis, the abnormal thickening and hardening of the arterial walls that can restrict the blood flow to the penis and keep it from getting firm enough to penetrate. Prosthetic implants, vacuum erection devices (VEDs), self-injectable vasoactive drugs such as papaverine and prostaglandin-E1, and the oral erectile dysfunction agents can be helpful.

I want to reiterate the important distinction between the type of patients for whom I do and do not recommend prosthetic devices and injectable medications. A typically acceptable candidate is the man who is suffering from the "leisure world syndrome." He is often a widower in his late sixties or seventies who starts to meet older women and begins to date. To his surprise, these women expect a level of sexual activity that he did not anticipate. He is not necessarily able to handle the challenge. This type of patient was usually not very sexually active in the latter years of his marriage, and now, for the first time in years, he is called upon to perform. This kind of patient is a legitimate candidate for a prosthetic implant or vasoactive injections, but generally only if he has not responded well to the oral medications (Viagra, Cialis, Levitra, Staxyn, or Stendra).

On the other end of the spectrum is an aging man who has been married for many years to the same woman. The couple has had a fulfilling life together and remain very much in love, even though their sex life has diminished. When they do attempt to have sex, the man finds he is incapable of getting an erection. He decides he wants his old sex life back again and comes to me for help. If I feel he is seeking treatment in the vain hope that it will restore his youthful vigor and virility, I do not encourage implants or vasoactive injections. If the couple has already adjusted to the absence of sex, these aggressive treatments are not advised. I have found that, once the novelty wears off, this man usually discontinues using the devices. Each case has to be evaluated on an individual basis, preferably with the partner involved in the decision. Treatment has done much good for some marriages of fifty years and longer.

Sex in the New Millennium

Based on my clinical experience and my understanding of current research, I am convinced that the future bodes well for the sex lives of people now entering their senior years and even better for those now middle-aged. I base this prediction on the burgeoning cultural view that the elderly can be active and fulfilled, even when it comes to sex, and on the amazing progress that has been made in extending the capacities of other bodily functions. In sports, what were once considered insurmountable barriers, such as the four-minute mile and the seven-foot high jump, now are accomplished routinely. The peak years of athletes have been dramatically extended. There is no reason why the years of active sexuality cannot be similarly extended.

Chapter 10

Sexually Transmitted Diseases

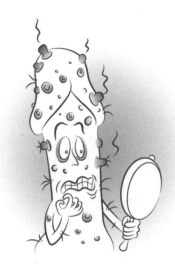

Let us hold off for a minute on what should be your primary concern—HIV/AIDS—and talk about the sexually transmitted diseases (STDs) that have faded from the spotlight over the past few years but remain a major public health challenge throughout the world. While significant progress has been made in preventing, diagnosing, and treating certain STDs, the Centers for Disease Control and Prevention (CDC) estimates that twenty million new infections occur each year in the United States alone.[1] The good news is that, when diagnosed properly, most STD infections can be treated. In many cases, once the symptoms are gone, they have no deleterious effect on penis power.

Chlamydia: Silent but Troublesome

Chlamydia, a bacterial infection, remains the most commonly reported infectious disease in the United States. More than 2.8 million new cases are estimated to occur each year.[2] Chlamydia is usually asymptomatic, meaning it rarely shows or produces indications of a disease or medical condition and therefore often goes undiagnosed. Untreated, it can cause severe health consequences for women, including pelvic inflammatory disease and ectopic pregnancy in which a fertilized egg is implanted outside the uterus, more than 95 percent of the time settling in the fallopian tubes. An ectopic pregnancy can cause fetal death and present grave dangers for the mother. Permanent damage to reproductive organs is probable.

Many gynecologists also report that chlamydia is one of the leading causes of infertility in women, and women infected with chlamydia are up to five times more likely to become infected with HIV, if exposed.[3] The chlamydia organism is responsible for nearly 40 percent of all recurring vaginal infections that do not respond to traditional treatment. In men, it can cause epididymitis, an inflammation or infection of the epididymis (a duct located on the posterior surface of the testicle), resulting in pain and swelling of the testicle. Chlamydia can also cause nonspecific urethritis, an inflammation of the male urethra. Even without symptoms, the infection can still be transmitted. Symptoms are likely to include a watery discharge and burning when you urinate. A simple urine test can detect chlamydia, and the organism can then be effectively treated with antibiotics.

Gonorrhea: This Clap Is Not a Cheer

The second most reported genital infectious disease in the United States is gonorrhea, often called the clap, a nickname that refers to a treatment in which the penis would be "clapped" on both sides simultaneously to clear the blockage in the urethra from gonorrhea pus. This primitive treatment for gonorrhea is no longer used but the name remains.

A national gonorrhea control program was implemented in the mid-1970s, and the rate of the disease declined 74 percent between 1975 and 1997. After several years with no further decline, rates began to drop again and reached their lowest levels in 2009. However, gonorrhea remains a highly infectious disease and a major global health problem.[4]

An infected patient usually comes in with a yellowish and pus-like discharge from the penis. While gonorrhea is easily cured, untreated cases can lead to serious health problems. Like chlamydia, gonorrhea in women is a major cause of pelvic inflammatory disease.

In men, untreated gonorrhea can cause chronic epididymitis and, more significantly, can involve the urethra and the prostate, causing severe scarring and lifelong strictures (abnormal narrowing in the urethra). Like chlamydia, studies suggest that the presence of gonorrhea makes an individual three to five times more likely to acquire HIV, if exposed. Fortunately, gonorrhea can usually be cured with oral or injected antibiotics. Drug resistance, however, is becoming an increasingly important concern and is especially worrisome among men who have sex with men, where resistance is eight times higher than among heterosexuals.

Syphilis: Next to AIDS, the Worst of All

Syphilis is a genital ulcerative disease that usually begins with a simple sore on the penis. If diagnosed early and treated with appropriate antibiotics, the sores will usually disappear. If the initial diagnosis is missed, the infection can linger without symptoms and develop into *secondary* syphilis, characterized by painful and highly contagious open sores. Congenital syphilis can cause stillbirth, death soon after birth, and physical deformity and neurological complications in children who survive. In adults, untreated syphilis can infect the central nervous system, causing paralysis, insanity, blindness, or death.

Untreated syphilis is rare today. But like many other STDs, syphilis facilitates the spread of HIV, increasing transmission of the viruses at least two- to fivefold. The rate of primary and secondary syphilis decreased throughout the 1990s. In 2000, it reached an all-time low. Alarmingly, between 2000 and 2005, a dramatic (81 percent) increase of infection for primary and secondary syphilis was seen among men, particularly those having unprotected sex with other men.[5] This subgroup of men is primarily responsible for the overall increase in the national syphilis rate. Syphilis rates have continued to increase overall between 2005 and 2014.[6]

Genital Herpes: Not the Scourge of the Twenty-First Century

Even more common is genital herpes. Approximately fifty million people in America are infected by the virus, and approximately 30 percent of adults carry the antibody.[7] Herpes can lie dormant for long periods of time, only to break out in blister-like lesions on the penis, especially during periods of stress, exhaustion, or illness. Symptoms might also include fever, headache, a burning sensation while urinating, and discharge. When the blisters appear, the infection is highly contagious. To a healthy male, the herpes blisters are virtually harmless, although they can be uncomfortable. They can be treated with topical ointments or oral medication and usually clear up completely in five to seven days. Herpes is a minor thorn in the side of a sexually active man—no more virulent than the common herpes blister on the lip (usually called a cold sore). Although herpes is *not* curable, or even preventable, in almost all instances it is no more than a transient annoyance in healthy men and women whose immune systems are intact.

Be Alert—It's Everywhere and It's Elusive

Human papilloma virus (HPV) is the most common sexually transmitted virus in the United States. About 79 million people in the country are currently infected, and about 14 million more get infected each year.[8]

HPV can cause unsightly warts that look like tiny cauliflowers on the genitals. The virus is highly contagious. Most of these lesions are removed with a topical application of a weak, vinegar-like chemical (urologists call it the pickle wrap). Stubborn growths might require electrocautery, liquid nitrogen freezing, or laser ablation. Once acquired, HPV can remain invisible and dormant and, similar to herpes, can reappear throughout the life of an infected person. Evidence is mounting that HPV can cause cervical, vaginal, and vulvar cancer in women. Presently, there is an FDA-approved vaccine called Gardasil. It works against HPV types 6, 11, 16, and 18 and is recommended to be given to females between the ages of nine and twenty-six. In the gay community, HPV has been associated with anal cancer. It is incumbent upon any responsible man to be treated promptly and make his partner aware of his condition should he acquire HPV, and it is further recommended that all sexually active males between the ages of nine and twenty-six be vaccinated with Gardasil as well.

Recent data from the CDC show that fewer than half of girls—and even fewer boys—ages thirteen to seventeen have received all three recommended doses of the HPV vaccine series, even though the vaccination has the potential to prevent up to three out of four HPV-associated cancers.[9] Remember, the only 100 percent effective way to prevent HPV infections is by not having sex! Get vaccinated.

AIDS: *The* Scourge of the Twenty-First Century

Genital infections can definitely cramp your style, and no responsible man should engage in sex if it means infecting his partner. Some STDs can cause temporary loss of libido and diminished capacity to obtain an erection, but with the notable exception of AIDS, all the commonly sexually transmitted infections are either curable or self-limited.

Acquired immune deficiency syndrome (AIDS) is a very different story. The virus that causes AIDS, human immunodeficiency virus (HIV), is found in bodily fluids and attacks the cells of the immune system, leaving the body so vulnerable to bacteria, viruses, and parasites that the outcome is almost invariably death. So far no known cure for AIDS exists, but the development of highly effective treatment regimens is prolonging the life of HIV-positive patients far beyond what we were capable of doing even fifteen years ago.

While the two most susceptible groups remain homosexual men and intravenous drug users, the incidence among heterosexuals is rising. Though heterosexuals face a greater statistical risk of dying from drunk driving or not wearing seat belts, as Magic Johnson's dramatic announcement in 1991 demonstrated, nobody is above the risk of HIV infection. Despite his robust survival, the infection and deaths of many other celebrity figures since that time have reinforced that this is not the age for casual sex with strangers. Superpotent men who are not in long-term relationships must recognize that when you have sex with someone, you are in a sense sleeping with everyone with whom that person has had sex.

As of this writing, the CDC in Atlanta recommends that people protect themselves by limiting their number of sexual partners, never sharing needles, and using condoms correctly and consistently.[10] Unfortunately, the lines of AIDS demarcation are increasingly difficult to define. For example, a woman, even though not an intravenous drug user, can nonetheless be infected with HIV from a sexual partner who is an intravenous drug user. She can then, in turn, transmit the virus to her subsequent sexual partners. They, in turn, can pass it on to their partners and so on—less like the domino effect and more like a fission explosion. That is what has happened in Africa and around the world!

Remember that the entire template of a partner's *prior* sexual experience will be permanently tattooed upon you. Those cultures or subcultures that encourage multiple sexual partners greatly facilitate the spread of HIV. The connection between AIDS and anal and oral sex has classically been implicated as the primary route of spread (excluding contaminated needles and blood products). Fellatio by itself *can* transmit HIV. The deadly virus can, in fact, find its way into your bloodstream through any minor break or crack, either in your skin or in the mucous membranes lining any body cavity.

Since there is no cure, extreme caution in both your choice of sexual partners and your sexual menu becomes your only defense. Knowing that your partner has passed an AIDS test is not enough, as the virus can be transmitted before it shows up in a test. In addition, you should heed the usual advice about using condoms or avoiding intercourse. I know condoms may cramp your style (some patients compare it to taking a shower with their socks on). I know sex feels a lot better without them. But your life is at stake. You can love sex even with latex. If you play by the new ground rules, you can still exercise your penis power to your heart's content. You just have to do it with discernment, caution, and care.

Chapter 11

What Women Need to Know

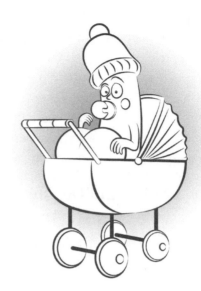

Some say that the way to a man's heart is through his stomach. While that may be true, in my opinion, the way to a man's *soul* is through his penis.

If I had my way, every woman would be a walking encyclopedia of penis knowledge, a wizard at enhancing penis power. My advice to women is to learn how, why, when, and where the penis works. Find out what your partner's penis needs, what it likes, what excites it. Cater to his penis, and it will cater to you.

I know some women will think this sounds sexist, but I assure you, I am in total support of equality in every aspect of life. I am not advocating for women to be subservient or to submit to any form of abuse or degradation. What I do advise is that women make their men's sexual satisfaction a high priority *for selfish reasons*. Make *him* happy, and he will make *you* happy. Give *to* him, and you are more likely to get what you want *from* him. A principle of human interaction is that we please other people because we want them to treat us well. The golden rule is never more powerful than when applied to the penis: "Do unto him as you wish he would do unto you."

I spend a great deal of time advising men to learn how to satisfy the women in their lives, but I believe women understand the give-and-take principle instinctively. Over the years, hundreds of women have asked me what they can do to enhance their partner's penis power. They might stammer or conjure up euphemisms, but they always want to know the secrets for improving their man's sexuality. I have never met a woman who did not want a superpotent man because I have never met a woman who did not want to be satisfied herself.

Ladies and Gentlemen: It Begins with Communication

If the man in your life does not openly let you know what he likes sexually, you can forget about it, experiment, or straight out ask him what he likes. Any sexual ignorance between you and your partner will only have harmful effects on your sex life, so I discourage the first choice. Learning what turns your partner on and delivering it as best you can is the most effective way to improve your partner's penis power. You can experiment by trying different strategies. If your man is not the expressive type, his answers might not be obvious, so it is important to experiment, and this invariably adds to the variety of your experience. I strongly recommend talking to him specifically about *his* needs, his desires, and even his fantasies. By asking him what *he* likes, you let him know you care about his happiness.

Some men are uncomfortable with candid sex talk. If that is the case in your situation, you might use a magazine article as a starting point: "I read that some men like . . ." You can also learn while making love and asking, "Do you like this?" or "Was that good?" He only has to grunt a response, and you will gather important information.

Communication is a two-way street, so you also want to make sure he understands *your* likes and dislikes. Talk openly, but remember, men have delicate egos, especially when it pertains to their penises. If you want your man to improve his lovemaking abilities, avoid saying anything that could be taken as a put-down, especially *while* making love. To correct or change his behavior, do it delicately and with compassion, as you would with a child. Focus on what you would *like* him to do, not what he is doing wrong. If you do not like some of his techniques, try telling him what you would *rather* he do. Even delicate matters such as early ejaculation can be handled this way. Instead of saying, "Can't you learn to control yourself?" you might say, "Making love to you is so wonderful. Wouldn't it be great if we could do it even longer? Let's work on it together." If you say anything that makes him feel defensive, it will surely increase his self-doubt, and self-doubt leads to performance anxiety and, eventually, penis failure. Try not to come across as overly demanding or intimidating. If you say (or even imply), "Shape up or else!" even a superpotent man might not rise to the occasion.

When your man does something you like, or if he shows any sign of trying to comply with your wishes, let him know you like it right away. Let him know you appreciate the effort, even if you have to exaggerate to get that positive message across. The slightest sign of pleasure from you will reinforce his confidence, which will, in turn, boost his penis power.

Women's Top Ten Complaints

In addition to the obvious problems—"He loses his erections at the worst times" and "He ejaculates prematurely"—both of which are discussed at great length elsewhere in this book, I hear the following complaints repeatedly from women.

"He wants to have sex when I'm not in the mood."

Men typically want sex more often than women, and many men expect their women to deliver on demand. Respect and consideration should be the top priority for anyone in an intimate relationship, and a smart woman might consider doing everything possible to enable her man to exercise his penis power. Naturally, saying no is sometimes appropriate, but by the same token, sometimes it is appropriate to say yes, even if you are not in the mood. In a good relationship, compromise is crucial. Every couple has to work out their own ground rules. In general, a woman who wants a happy, healthy man will try to be there for him. The ultimate beneficiary of your generosity will be you.

"Sometimes he turns me down when I want him."

Most men love it when a woman initiates sex, and they love being seduced, but an overly aggressive woman can threaten a man. It's important to find balance. Of course, some men, especially those who are more conservative, *hate* it when women initiate sex. These men feel it is a man's place to "get things rolling." Try every weapon in your arsenal, but if he continues to be a reluctant lover, it might be a sign of deeper problems in the relationship.

His hesitancy might also be due to something completely unrelated to your relationship. He might be stressed by work. In such cases, try doing what his business associates do when they want his attention: make an appointment. Rent a hotel room near his office if you must—a great way to rekindle the romance!

"He's so businesslike when we make love!"

When a man is sexually charged and ready to go, his animal instincts take over, and gone is the playfulness, the passion of the ardent lover, sweet words, grace, and charm. The truth is, if you are looking for a lover with the elegance and smoothness of James Bond, you might have to rethink your expectations. On the other hand, if you want a man who can have fun while making love, you have a good chance of making changes. Many men get overly serious because they are nervous about their performance. Lead the way to laughter by making him feel as comfortable as possible. As for whispering in your ear and telling you he loves you, if you do it first, and he cannot return the sentiment, talk with him *after* you make love. Teaching passion and romance is hard, but a satisfied man might be willing to work on his manners.

"Sometimes he does things that hurt me."

I hear two kinds of complaints from women in this regard. The first has to do with clumsy or rough behavior during foreplay: "He bites my nipples like they are cookies," or "He rubs my clitoris like he's polishing his car." Men in the throes of sexual passion can become insensitive to their partner's physical and emotional feelings. In addition, some men develop crude habits when they first start having sex, and unfortunately, nobody has ever smoothed out those rough spots. A man might actually think you *like* what he is doing. He may have known women who *did*. You absolutely must let him know if he is hurting you. Do not let his missteps ruin your experience. Tell him gently, so he does not take it as criticism or a sign of failure. If after you talk to him, he continues to ignore your requests, and if you choose not to end the relationship, a more serious reprimand is appropriate. Any woman who finds herself in a sexually abusive relationship should seek counseling or distance herself from that man until he makes serious changes in his behavior.

The other kind of pain occurs during intercourse and includes too much internal friction (which might be solved by a vaginal lubricant), thrusting too hard against the pubic bone, awkwardly yanking or twisting the body, or leaning his weight on a tender spot. You have to help him change his habits. One source of pain is biologically determined, and that is a penis that is too big. Unfortunately, no medical solution can fix this. The answer is to adjust the angle of penetration and depth of insertion until you find a combination that is both satisfying and comfortable. No rule says a penis has to penetrate to its full length. Communication and experimentation are the best solutions.

"He wants me to do things I find distasteful."

Both partners in a relationship should respect each other's limitations and uphold each other's values. Establishing personal boundaries is essential for any intimate relationship.

If you are a woman who dislikes oral sex, you should not feel ashamed of your reluctance. On the other hand, examine your resistance—nothing is inherently dangerous, dirty, or evil about oral sex. Many women find it stimulating, especially if they are madly in love with their partners and enjoy bringing them pleasure.

Your aversion may be to swallowing semen. If so, you might have to negotiate, offering to do it only until he is ready to ejaculate. Also, no rule says you can't spit out his semen, though you should know there is no danger in swallowing semen unless it is infected. Semen is not a waste product. Quite the contrary, it is the most vital fluid in the male body. Without it, human life would be extinct.

If your partner makes other sexual demands from you that you find distasteful, such as anal sex, uncomfortable positions, or sex in strange places or times, the best solution is to communicate your aversion. After speaking openly, he should be willing to change, and if he is unwilling or persists, you may want to seek professional counseling.

"My husband is a wham-bam-thank-you-ma'am kind of guy, and all he knows is the missionary position."

The simple solution is to educate him! In a gentle way, let him know that you so enjoy being intimate that you would like to savor the experience by slowing down. You can ask, "What's the rush?" Teach him that an extra few minutes of loving foreplay or passionate intercourse will bring *both* of you heightened pleasure.

Keep in mind that sometimes men's instincts take over, even if their minds are screaming, "Slow down!" If such occurrences are the *exception*, you should be able to tolerate it from time to time, even if it means that only one of you leaves the bed satisfied. This does not mean you should tolerate crude or thoughtless behavior. If the "quickie" is the norm, asking him to modify his in-bed behavior can be the best way to initiate change.

If your man has a limited imagination, lend him yours. Make explicit suggestions. If that does not work, make him an offer he cannot refuse.

"My lover does not want me to touch his penis."

This is not a common problem but occurs most often in new relationships and usually stems from either a man's fear of premature ejaculation or an abnormal, deep-rooted fear of being touched. The first scenario usually improves as soon as the man feels secure in his performance. The second is more intractable and takes patience. I recommend gradual steps to make him comfortable with the idea of being fondled. Start by stroking his penis with one finger for a short amount of time or rubbing it with your thigh or arm, and work your way gradually to normal manual stimulation. Treat his reluctant penis with kid gloves until his fears dissipate.

"Sometimes he annoys me so much I cannot bring myself to have sex with him, even though I'm feeling sexual."

Every couple has their conflicts, and all individuals have their own set of pet peeves. The secret to making an intimate relationship last is to find a way to ignore what you cannot change. If the rift is serious, by all means work it out, either privately or with a counselor. If your relationship is thrown off track by run-of-the-mill irritations, do yourself a favor, and do not let that get in the way of sex. When the infamous bank robber Willie Sutton was asked why he robbed banks, he replied, "Because that's where the money is," which led to Danoff's law: "Satisfy your man's penis because that's where his soul is." After a good roll in the hay, you will have worked off that frustration, and your man will be much more amenable to sympathizing with your grievances and working toward a resolution.

"When my husband has a few drinks, all he wants to do is have sex, but I don't like him in that condition."

If your man needs a little booze to lower his inhibitions, it is not necessarily bad. Unfortunately, many women tell me that too much alcohol turns an amorous man into a clumsy, insensitive brute and also keeps his penis from reaching the launching pad. Again this requires diplomacy. Tell him why you prefer to make love when he *has not* been drinking. Make sure you have the conversation with him when he is sober. If your partner has a serious drinking or drug problem, one that is a threat to his own health and is causing problems in your love life, recommend he seek professional treatment immediately.

"I'm a single mother. How can I educate my son about penis power?"

Provide your son with unconditional love, and let him know at every possible opportunity that he's worthy of self-respect. If you raise a healthy, self-assured son, chances are he will feel secure in his penis image. You can provide him with facts as easily as a man can, but you cannot speak from experience and thus cannot be a role model. A male relative or close male friend that you and your son trust can teach him about his body and sexuality and thus compensate to some degree for the absence of a father. If the surrogate is a man of true superpotency, his presence might serve your son's penis education better than a real father who is not around.

Penis-Oriented Women Have More Fun

I encourage women who still have unanswered questions to do everything in their power to become as well educated as possible in all matters pertaining to the penis. A woman who is penis oriented is also empowered to create her own happiness and to have more fun, a better marriage, a more faithful husband, a happier home, and greater personal fulfillment. If women spent as much time attending to their men's penises as they devote to their hair, makeup, and clothing, they would get more of what they want and have far more satisfying relationships.

Being penis oriented does *not* make you less than an equal to the man in your life and does not require sacrificing your intelligence or self-respect. It simply means learning to understand and accommodate a man's penis needs by approaching that task with all the pride and skill that you would bring to any endeavor. Based on my decades of clinical experience, if you take the steps to become informed, you and your man will reap rewards you have only dreamed about.

Chapter 12

Penis
FAQs

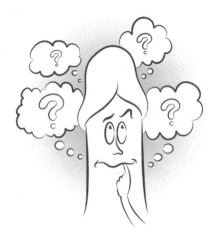

This chapter addresses some of the questions that I am frequently asked but that have not yet been fully covered elsewhere in this book.

Q: Do women prefer certain kinds of penises to others?

A: I have had thousands of conversations with women about the most intimate details of their sex lives, and they have told me details they have related to no other person. For the most part, women never seriously express to me a strong preference for one kind of penis over another. Believe me, I have asked! Some women do have a definite preference as to size or shape, but the overwhelming majority confess that length, width, appearance, and complexion do not matter in a long-term relationship.

The only real concerns I have heard are regarding what we call a micropenis, an abnormally small penis. The true micropenis is extremely rare. Ultimately, with the exception of those men who lie outside the middle of the curve, I stand by the belief that men can be as "big" as they think they are. The majority of partners care most about *hardness* and *responsiveness*; some mention cleanliness.

The penis is a functional organ, not necessarily an aesthetic object. For this reason, some women may require a larger functioning penis to stimulate them to orgasm. In most cases, this is simply an anatomical fact (a taller or larger woman will invariably have more body fat, creating a greater distance over which an erect penis must traverse, or a larger vagina that requires a larger penis for stimulation). Both partners should communicate their physical needs and personal desires. Experimenting with different positions and alternative or additional methods of stimulation can help satisfy both partners and go a long way toward maintaining a strong emotional and sexual relationship.

Knowledge is power, and the sexual power of a man can be elevated when he simply learns how to cater to the specific and unique needs of his partner. Ultimately, the penis, regardless of its size, is but one of many sexual tools men have at their disposal. The more you learn how to use your entire body to stimulate your partner, the less important one part of the body becomes.

Q: Is there a legitimate way to make my penis any larger?

A: The answer is unequivocally no! Surgeons have discovered and are using a number of techniques, including skin grafts (known as dermal matrix grafts), in an attempt to increase the girth of the penis. These procedures, as well as a lengthening technique that increases penis length by severing the suspensory ligaments, are falsely represented as legitimate ways to increase the size of the penis. Phalloplasty and lengthening procedures are inventions of hucksters, charlatans, and fakes. Not only ineffective, they are also highly risky.

Q: If I have sex a lot, can I damage my penis?

A: The chances of injuring your penis are miniscule, no matter how vigorously you exercise it. Nature has designed your penis to be able to take much more of a thrashing than most other appendages. With the exception of whales, no mammals have bones in their penises, although some mammals have an *os*, a bone-like appendage made of rigid connective tissue. In human males, the penis has no bones and so nothing to fracture. Nor are there ligaments, joints, or muscles to strain or tear. Surrounding the corpora cavernosa is a fibrous tunica, tissue so tough that I have to apply extreme pressure just to incise it when performing surgery. When the penis is erect and the corpora are filled with blood, a sharp blow or trauma could rupture the tunica. Such incidents are extremely rare and are mistakenly called a fractured penis. It is also possible to rupture the surface capillaries of the penis, causing discoloration and bruising. This is also unusual.

If you have heard any man complaining of a penis injury, chances are it had to do with the *skin*, the most vulnerable part of the penis, which can suffer abrasions, cuts, and bruises. These occur most often from accidents like getting your penis stuck in a zipper. The most frequent sex-related injury is skin irritation caused by excessive friction, and this keeps more men from having sex than any other injury and is why one of my colleagues believes that "lubricants have saved more marriages than Dear Abby." The glans (the head of the penis) can become bruised by thrusting against a woman's pubic bone or other hard body part. Again, traumatic injuries are more often caused by something *other* than ordinary sex.

Most of the penis injuries I see in my office and in the emergency room are self-inflicted. You would not believe the number of objects I have removed from penises—not just rings and clips that perforate the skin, but long, thin items inserted into the urethra, including pencils, pens, pins, wires, and especially swizzle sticks (drink mixers).

Q: If I use my penis a lot sexually, will it become weaker or "burn out" as I get older?

A: You have no predetermined number of orgasms, no quota of erections or ejaculations, and no upper limit that can be exceeded. Your seminal vesicles will not dry up if you ejaculate too much. Your penis will not become flaccid if you have sex a thousand times. You may get fatigued from having a lot of sex, just as you would from *any* physical activity, but if you use your penis frequently and vigorously, it will invigorate the rest of your body and keep your spirit young and vibrant. Penis *underuse* is a much bigger problem than *overuse*.

Q: I have a history of heart disease. Do I have to limit my sexual practices?

A: Every heart patient should be advised according to his specific condition and consult with his cardiologist prior to vigorous activity of any kind, including sex. However, I must dispel the myth that having sex is damaging to the heart. In the past, men who survived heart attacks were often told not to have sex, and they were also told not to exercise and to retire from physically demanding work. We now know that, within appropriate limits, exercise is good for heart patients. Sex is no different. Not only is it a terrific form of exercise, but also it is unsurpassed in lifting the spirit of a man who has suffered the trauma of a heart attack. I must, however, issue an important caveat. If you have a history of heart disease, you should not be overdoing *anything*, including sex. As with any form of exercise, if you get chest pain while having sex, stop immediately and see your cardiologist as soon as possible. I frequently see older men with cardiovascular problems experiencing delayed ejaculation. Because it takes them longer to reach climax, these men get caught up in a frenzy of exertion, aiming for the elusive orgasm. If you are an older man and have experienced cardiovascular problems, take your time during sex. If you do not recognize your limits and adjust your practices accordingly, dire consequences can ensue.

One other caution: if you suffer from coronary artery disease and have occasional exertion-related chest pain (angina) and you treat the pain with nitroglycerin, you should *never* take any of the oral medications for erectile dysfunction. Each of these PDE-5 inhibitors is a potent vasodilator and in combination with nitroglycerin (also a potent vasodilator) can cause a fatal drop in blood pressure.

Q: Is it possible to become addicted to sex?

A: From a medical standpoint, the answer is no. Our criterion for addiction is based on the presence of physiological symptoms of withdrawal. Being deprived of sex does not feel good, and different men will suffer to a lesser or greater extent, but that does not constitute addiction any more than suffering over a lack of food makes you a food addict or feeling restless because you have not worked out makes you an exercise junkie. Like food and exercise, sex is nonaddictive.

Men can become *compulsive* about or *obsessed* with sex. In extreme cases, this can impact negatively on other aspects of life. Sexual obsession is not caused by too much sexual activity. It usually is a function of deep-rooted psychological problems, and men with that condition should seek consultation with a qualified psychotherapist.

Q: If I take testosterone, will I become a better lover?

A: As discussed in chapter 9, unless your testosterone level is abnormally low to begin with, taking supplementary testosterone by injection or topical application will not change your ability to get or keep an erection, nor will it improve your sexual capacity in any way. In fact, taking excessive amounts of testosterone can be physically detrimental.

Q: My friends seem to be more interested in sex than I am. Is there something wrong with me?

A: Levels of desire vary widely among men. One study of college students had the subjects press a counter every time they had a sexual thought or fantasy. Some students clicked more than three hundred times a day, while others reported they rarely had a sexual thought.[1] What's important is that you are personally able to satisfy whatever level of sexual desire you have. If you have a paucity of interest in pursuing sexual encounters or are too afraid or too busy to engage in romance, take the time to examine the reasons. If you feel intimidated by sex because of bad experiences in the past, follow the advice I have outlined throughout this book. Think positively. Move forward.

Q: I am thinking of having a vasectomy. Will it affect my penis power?

A: Vasectomy is a safe, effective method of birth control for men who no longer wish to have children. The procedure involves interrupting the continuity of the vas deferens, the tube that carries sperm from the testicles, where sperm is made, to the seminal vesicles, where sperm is stored until ejaculation. Basically, vasectomy stops only the passage of sperm, so that none of it is included in the semen you ejaculate. The procedure itself is performed in less than ten minutes in a doctor's office under a local anesthesia through a tiny nick in the scrotal skin (the "no scalpel" technique). The postoperative discomfort is minimal and rarely requires analgesics.

As for penis power, a vasectomy causes no reduction in sensation, no lowering of desire, no less circulating testosterone, no loss of ability to get or keep an erection, and no less satisfaction when having an orgasm. The only difference after a vasectomy is that you release no sperm. Sperm comprises a miniscule portion of the seminal fluid, so there is no reduction in the volume of semen ejaculated.

For many men, a vasectomy has the potential to increase penis power because they are no longer inhibited by concerns about pregnancy. Long-time partners often feel more spontaneous. They do not have to interrupt lovemaking to deal with diaphragms or condoms, and they often feel heightened sensations during intercourse because there is no latex between the penis and the vagina.

Some vasectomy patients change their minds about having children and request a reversal, a vasovasostomy, which involves reconnecting the vas deferens. This is a more difficult procedure than the original vasectomy but has a high rate of success, and most patients are able to conceive children afterward. Just as with a vasectomy, the reversal does not diminish penis power. In fact, there is a potential bonus: after a vasovasostomy, a couple is now making love with the express purpose of conceiving a child. Lovemaking is often more romantic than ever.

Q: Are there any other alternatives for male birth control?

A: Unfortunately, no effective and practical alternatives for male birth control exist at this point other than abstinence, a vasectomy, the use of condoms or other prophylactics, or withdrawal. With the rapid rate of advances we have seen in medical science, I predict men will soon be able to simply take a pill to control the release of sperm, just as some women take a pill to control the release of their eggs.

Q: I heard that a "cock ring" would help me last longer before ejaculating. Do you recommend the use of such a device?

A: No. In the hope of prolonging intercourse, some men place metallic or elastic constriction rings around the base of their penises after an erection is achieved. Theoretically, the ring impedes the venous outflow, so the blood trapped within the penis shaft cannot escape, and the penis stays erect longer. It sounds good in principle, but it can be dangerous. There is a danger of blood sludging or clotting or even rupture of the delicate sinusoids of the penis. When blood is trapped in the penis and cannot escape, a persistent and painful erection known as priapism can form. The damage can sometimes be irreversible.

If you want to delay ejaculation, you are better off trying some of the techniques described in chapters 7 and 15.

Q: Ever since my wife gave birth, I do not feel like having sex. What is happening?

A: Surveys indicate this is common. One theory holds that postnatal changes in a woman's body might make her less attractive to her husband. Another possibility is that the demands of parenting can wear down a mother and exhaust a father. In my mind, the main reason is that after giving birth, the wife's attention shifts dramatically from her mate to her child. It is normal and natural for a mother's energy to be focused on her baby. Unfortunately, even men who share that sense and appreciate their wives' commitment to the child might, on some unconscious level, feel rejected and require psychological adjustments and modifications in the timing and circumstances of lovemaking. It is crucial to understand the dynamics at work and not to interpret your wife's behavior as a form of rejection.

Q: I want sex a lot more than my partner does. What can I do about that?

A: About one-third of the couples seeking marital or relationship help do so because of a marked discrepancy in desire levels. This common problem is reflected in the old joke: What do you call foreplay in a marriage? Answer: begging.

No man likes to be rejected or to beg for sex. On average, men have higher levels of desire than women and find themselves in the mood for sex more often than women. Unfortunately, if you suppress your sexual frustration, you run the risk of becoming hostile and resentful, and you might stop initiating sex altogether rather than face the possibility of rejection. And, of course, you might be tempted to look elsewhere for sex.

A superpotent man should do everything in his power to fulfill his sexual needs, and a partner who responds with enthusiasm each and every time he wants to have sex is ideal. In reality, coaxing, cajoling, and all forms of seduction might have to be employed, and even some subtle forms of bribery (jewelers and florists can attest to that). No one should be reduced to actual begging, although I have a surprisingly large number of patients who are not above pleading. When approached with a sense of humor, even that may be justified. Superpotent men are pragmatic: they do whatever it takes to get the job done.

The best approach is to talk openly and candidly about your needs and about the discrepancies in your desire levels. If two people care enough about satisfying each other's needs, they can usually overcome the complications caused by a difference in levels of desire. If your efforts fail, it may be time to see a counselor.

Q: Why do I seem to have more penis power in the summer?

A: When it comes to superpotency, hot is better than cold. That is why most couples honeymoon in Hawaii and not the Klondike. Tropical flowers, scented air, and hula dancers create a seductive ambience, but so do the physical effects of warmth. Have you noticed what happens to your scrotum when you plunge into a cold pool? The skin contracts drastically, the scrotal sac shrinks to the size of a peanut, and the testicles retract into the inguinal canal. Cold also causes vasoconstriction, or narrowing of the blood vessels. None of these conditions is conducive to penis power.

So why all the partying in frigid ski resorts? After an invigorating day on the slopes, the fireplace, hot tub, or a thick down comforter feel downright tropical.

Q: My orgasms are not as explosive as they used to be, and I do not release as much semen. Is something wrong?

A: This is a common question. Invariably, the men asking it are in their forties (if they are older, they have usually been carrying the question around for a while). As men age, their bodies produce less seminal fluid, and the volume of ejaculate decreases. This is normal and natural. The volumetric rule in urology states that ejaculatory volume (semen) is inversely proportional to advancing age. In lay terms, this means that the older men get, the less ejaculatory volume they have. This rule also applies to the frequency of intercourse (the older one gets and the more frequently one has intercourse, the smaller the ejaculatory volume becomes). Semen volume is inversely proportional to frequency. The refractory period also changes proportionally with age: the older men get, the longer the refractory period becomes. Why do your orgasms feel less intense? You still enjoy your favorite food, but eating it the hundredth time does not compare to the intensity of previous meals. The more substantive reason for diminished intensity can be found in the complex associations created by your mind.

Q: Is there any way to make my orgasms last longer?

A: This is one area where men are jealous of women. I call it Venus envy. For whatever reason, nature designed humans so that women can have prolonged wavelike orgasms while men can have brief and thunderous orgasms, five to seven seconds in duration. Men dream of making that ecstatic sensation last a full minute, five minutes, or an hour. So far, we have found ways to *delay* orgasm, but not to *prolong* it. (I am told that the Indian tradition of tantric yoga teaches esoteric techniques for extending sexual ecstasy, but I cannot vouch for this.)

I do predict that we will find a way to prolong male orgasm somehow, someday.

Q: Do superpotent men masturbate?

A: Masturbation is normal and should not elicit any form of shame or embarrassment. However, it should be the last resort for the superpotent man. Every man is alone at times, and under such circumstances, masturbation is certainly better than no sexual activity. I believe men who cannot go through a day without servicing themselves or who are obsessed with watching pornography need to reexamine their view of sex. Pornography not only presents a completely unrealistic view of sex in general but also has the potential to instill unhealthy habits. Masturbation is no substitute for sex, and too much masturbation can increase self-doubt. Mutual masturbation is another matter entirely. Couples who know how to use their hands and fingers with the artistry of violinists can fill a bedroom with fantastically erotic music.

Q: Does circumcision affect penis power?

A: No scientifically controlled experiments have been done regarding the sexual performance of circumcised versus uncircumcised men. Based upon my clinical experience, there is no difference. Some people assume that the circumcised man has greater sensitivity because he has no foreskin covering the glans. Others believe that the uncircumcised man has greater sensitivity because he has a foreskin. Neither is true.

The fact is that the foreskin retracts when an uncircumcised man has an erection, so in the aroused state, the penises are virtually the same.

Q: Is it wise to circumcise a newborn?

A: Uncircumcised men have a vastly greater chance of getting penile cancer. Cancer of the penis, which is rare, is virtually unheard of among circumcised men. Recent studies of AIDS prevention in Africa suggest that male circumcision can reduce the chance of HIV in men and perhaps in women. The validity of this is still being tested, but research shows that the cells on the underside of the foreskin are prime targets for the virus; tears and abrasions in the foreskin serve as an easy port of entry for the retrovirus. Other studies have estimated that circumcised men have a 44 to 60 percent lower risk for HIV infection.[2] Although this research is still evolving, it is fair to conclude that circumcision for men should be promoted at least with regard to HIV prevention.

Also, if an uncircumcised man does not regularly retract the foreskin and wash underneath it, the natural secretions from the skin can produce a smelly, cheesy substance known as smegma, which can lead to irritation, pain, and even infection.

Generally speaking, circumcision remains a healthier choice, but it has no effect on penis power, and I do not recommend it for my adult uncircumcised patients unless a medical problem warrants it, such as persistent irritation, infection, rash, or the inability to retract the foreskin for cleaning. Another legitimate reason for circumcision is if a man's sexual partner requests that he have one as a matter of personal preference. Adult circumcision is quick, simple, and safe when performed by an experienced and qualified urologist.

Q: My doctor says I must have surgery for prostate cancer. I am afraid I will become impotent. Is there any alternative?

A: I had a patient named Morton, a widower in his sixties who had recently married a beautiful, bright woman in her forties. Morton was having the time of his life when we found a malignant tumor in his prostate. Given his age and the nature and extent of his cancer, the treatment with the greatest likelihood of cure was the surgical removal of his prostate. I told Morton the truth: we could be reasonably certain of curing his cancer, but we could not give a 100 percent guarantee that his ability to get satisfactory erections would be preserved. It was a choice between risking the spread of cancer and potentially risking partial loss of his potency.

Morton was so terrified at the thought of losing perhaps 10 percent of the firmness of his erections that he insisted on an alternative treatment. I recommended the most advanced nerve-sparing surgical procedure available, which uses the da Vinci laparoscopic robot. There would be no unsightly scar, and the magnification afforded by this technique would allow the most meticulous preservation of the nerves of potency available (see chapter 5 for more details on laparoscopic procedures). Instead of following my recommendation, Morton opted for a far less effective treatment because it promised less potential loss of penis power. Several years later, I learned that Morton was dying of metastatic prostate cancer. The disease that had started in his prostate was now widely disseminated. A brilliant and successful businessman with a reputation for making smart decisions, Morton had literally sacrificed his life by thinking with his penis instead of his brain.

Pay attention to your urologist. As medical doctors, we have vast clinical experience and years of training that enable us to sort out all the variables. Have your urologist explain exactly what your condition is and what the benefits and risks are with *each* of the alternative treatment methods that are applicable in your particular case. (See chapters 5 and 6 for more information about prostate cancer treatment methods and options for counteracting any loss of penis power.)

Q: As a father, what can I do to help my son grow up to be a super-potent man?

A: You are your son's primary penis role model. The smallest message from you—a nod, a grunt, a shrug, a casual remark—gets carved into his memory more deeply than anything he picks up in a sex-education class or on the schoolyard. Set a good, responsible example with a *super-potent* attitude. A father who keeps his genitals under cover all the time, never mentions the word *penis*, or avoids his son's questions about sexuality will raise a self-conscious and probably self-doubting son. If you are open and honest and demonstrate penis pride, your son will absorb the right education.

You can reinforce your example by being candid and up-front about penis matters without making too big a deal about it. Treat the penis as a fact of life, not as something dirty to be hidden behind a zipper or something of great mystery that cannot be spoken about in public. Boys are extremely curious about their penises. If they suppress their curiosity because their parents evade the topic, they will come of age in ignorance or get their penis education the wrong way—from their peers. Do not pull punches, hide behind euphemisms, or limit discussion to brief moments or offhand comments.

When my son turned seven, he asked me, "When will my penis be as big as yours?" I said, "Put your hand in mine. When your fingers are as long as mine, which they definitely will be, then your penis will be as big as my penis." I knew perfectly well that the penis is special (my son would not have bothered asking when his hands or feet would be as big as mine), but I treated the question casually. Of course, the mere fact that a son can ask that question suggests that he grew up in an atmosphere of openness. When boys go through puberty and adolescence, *all* of them wonder if their organ is normal. Let your son know that his penis is perfectly fine, and help build and reinforce his self-confidence by describing the unique qualities of the penis: that it is a pleasure-giving appendage that should be appreciated, respected, and used wisely.

When I was a teenager, I was self-conscious about being shorter than many girls at school, and one day after a party, I told my father that despite being popular and a good dancer I was embarrassed to ask girls taller than me to dance. My father responded with a big smile that let me know I was okay. Then he said, "You know, son, all girls are the same size lying down."

This simple man-to-man moment had a big impact on me, subtly instilling in me the confidence to approach *any* girl. (Later on, by the way, I learned that my father was somewhat right anatomically: there is relatively little size difference among most people if you measure from the pubic bone to the neck; the length of the legs primarily creates height differences. When you are horizontal for sexual purposes, height becomes irrelevant, except in extreme cases.)

One caveat: sexual candor does not entail prying into your child's life. Teenagers need privacy. Unnecessary pressure has no place in your relationship with your son. Some fathers think they are instilling positive sexual attitudes by sharing sexy books or movies or alluding to their own exploits. Do not defeat your purpose by creating standards that make your child apprehensive and uncertain. Give your son the message that he and his penis are okay just the way they are. Superpotency is a matter of penis attitude, and penis attitude is a direct reflection of self-image. Teach your child to judge himself by his own standards, not by yours or anyone else's.

Q: What about bladder cancer and immunotherapy?

A: Bladder cancer is the second most common cancer of the urinary tract and accounts for about 7 percent of all new cases of cancer in men and 2 percent in women.[3] It is primarily a disease of senior citizens, and it is eminently treatable.

Early bladder cancer causes few if any symptoms and is almost always diagnosed after blood is seen in the urine, either under a microscope in a lab (microscopic hematuria) or in the toilet bowl.

The presence of blood in the urine mandates a visit to a urologist. The diagnosis is confirmed by use of a cystoscope, a fiber-optic camera that is easily inserted into the urinary bladder. If a bladder tumor is indeed identified, biopsies will be done on the spot to determine the type of tumor, its degree of aggressiveness, and penetration (if any) into the muscular wall of the urinary bladder.

The good news is that about 75 percent of these early tumors are localized and are easily treatable at the time of diagnosis and pose little risk of spreading beyond the confines of the urinary bladder.

Almost all early, noninvasive bladder tumors are treated endoscopically, where no skin incision is required to enter the bladder. The procedure is called TURBT (transurethral resection of bladder tumor). Once the pathologist has reviewed the biopsy material and ensures the urologist that the cancer has not invaded the bladder wall, the urologist will initially begin a program of active surveillance utilizing cystoscopic examinations on a periodic basis. Since bladder tumors are multifocal (they can appear anywhere in the bladder) and recurrent, meticulous follow-up is required.

Should one of these noninvasive bladder tumors recur, intravesical immunotherapy will usually be started. The most common immunotherapy agent instilled into the bladder is BCG (Bacillus Calmette-Guérin), a weakened strain of the tuberculosis bacillus. Although the exact mechanism by which BCG exerts its antitumor effect is not known, BCG does create an inflammatory reaction within the bladder, to which the patient responds dramatically, in its immune battle against disease.

The use of BCG immunotherapy significantly reduces the recurrence rate of these tumors, especially in patients who have high-risk, aggressive superficial bladder cancers.

Q: What can I do to prevent medical problems in my sexual organs?

A: Unfortunately, the average physician sadly neglects to examine male genitals. Most physical exams, other than those done by urologists, do not include even a cursory examination of the area. In most cases, physicians do not even ask questions about the patient's sex life, which could provide clues to physical disorders. This reality for men stands in stark contrast to the rigorous yearly exams most women undergo with their gynecologists and is a major contributing factor to the widespread ignorance I have witnessed in men with regard to awareness of their bodies in general and their genitals specifically.

For urologists, by far the most common male problem we see is enlargement of the prostate. All men over forty should insist on a digital rectal examination (which is not a computerized process, but rather a rectal exam done by the gloved finger or digit of the examining physician) when they have their physicals. While this procedure can be uncomfortable and embarrassing, it is a small price to pay for detecting the early warning signs of trouble. Early diagnosis of prostate cancer has an extremely high success rate of restoring prostate health. If a prostate cancer has not extended beyond the prostate, prompt, early treatment offers a high percentage of disease-free survival. If you experience any of the following symptoms, you should seek an immediate urologic consultation:

- A weak or interrupted urinary stream
- Difficulty starting the urinary stream
- The need to urinate frequently, especially throughout the night
- Blood in the urine
- Dribbling after you think you have completely emptied your bladder
- Painful or burning urination (dysuria)
- Persistent pain in the lower back, pelvis, or lower abdomen

Bear in mind that we now have many sophisticated, noninvasive tests for diagnosing prostate disease. Although a number of theories have attempted to explain how and why this deadly disease comes about, not enough scientific and medical evidence is available at this time to identify a definitive cause. Some studies have indicated that heredity is a major factor. For example, a man who has a blood relative who has had prostate cancer before turning sixty is twice as likely to develop the disease than the average man.[4] If a man has two blood relatives who have had the disease (for example, a father *and* a brother), the chances he will get the disease are at least four times greater.[5] Other studies have shown that the rate of incidence is also related to race. Prostate cancer has been found to be highest among African Americans and lowest among Asians. Surprisingly, studies show a low rate of incidence among Africans. Since African Americans share some genetic lineage with Africans, this difference suggests that dietary and lifestyle habits can play a role in the development of prostate cancer. Although much of this research is still in a preliminary phase, anecdotal evidence gives some indication that prostate cancer is related to both genes and lifestyle.

I have one suggestion in addition to regular examinations for preventing prostate problems: *have a lot of sex*. Like all organs, the prostate benefits from exercise, and the best exercise is ejaculation. When you ejaculate, your perineal muscles (the band of muscles that make up the perineum, the space between the rectum and the base of the testicle) contract violently. This provides a massage of sorts for the prostate gland, which keeps its ducts open and prevents its internal fluids from becoming stagnant.

New technology enables us to detect various tumors in the urinary bladder or testicles at an early stage. The treatment of testicular cancer has vastly improved over the past few years. In 1963, 63 percent of patients suffering from testicular cancer survived; now, more than 95 percent are curable.[6] Unlike prostate cancer, testicular cancer occurs mainly in men under forty. Regardless of your age, however, I strongly suggest that you self-examine your testicles monthly and feel for suspicious lumps (and also educate your male children). Just as doctors recommend that women (from teenage years on) examine their breasts for lumps to screen for breast cancer, men need to examine their testicles.

The best time for self-examination is after a warm bath or shower when the scrotum is relaxed. Your testicles should feel like hard-boiled eggs without the shells: smooth and void of lumps. Any lump, even a painless one, should be reported to your doctor immediately. You may palpate an abnormality during self-examination, or your sexual partner may notice it while making love. In either case, further evaluation by your urologist is a must. (Incidentally, if you notice that one of your testes is lower than the other, do not panic. One testis is *always* lower. It is nature's way of making sure those two sources of life do not crash into one another—a design for which all men should be grateful!)

Finally, if you ever experience a *sudden* onset of penis weakness, first rule out all possible *physical* causes by seeing a doctor immediately. If you do not have a doctor who examines your genitals, or if your doctor is someone with whom you are not comfortable discussing your sexual well-being, try to find one who understands that your sexual organs are not merely machines that perform biological services. A good doctor comprehends that the penis is not just a functional body part but also a psychological and spiritual agent designed to bring you pleasure.

Part 2

Becoming a Superpotent Man

Chapter 13

What's Your Penis Personality?

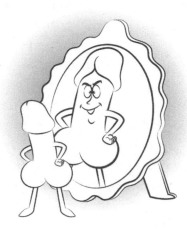

"It has a mind of its own" is one of those classic clichés I constantly hear from patients and friends in reference to their penises, reflecting the idea I call the penis mystique. One of the reasons we are so fascinated by that junior partner, as a lawyer patient of mine calls his, is that it *does* seem to think for itself. What other organ grows to several times its normal size, then shrinks again, sometimes despite our intentions and without warning? What other organ is so unpredictable? We often speak about it and even *to* it, as if it were a person. Men say, "My penis did this," as if it makes its own decisions. But however much your penis appears to act on its own, it does not have a mind of its own. On the contrary, it reads your mind, and your *heart* and *soul*. The behavior of your penis is an accurate reflection of your state of being, reflecting your thoughts and feelings more accurately than any other part of your body.

When you feel strong, vigorous, creative, and confident, your penis is strong, vigorous, creative, and confident, too. When you feel tired, apathetic, depressed, or impatient, your penis is, too. Even though you may not always be in touch with what you are thinking and feeling, your penis *is* in touch. Through a vast network of nerves and blood vessels, the penis has a direct connection to your brain. And you cannot fool it. Your penis will reveal your true feelings by its behavior.

If your partner offends you or hurts you, you can bet that, no matter how hard you try to conceal your feelings, your penis will act hurt and offended. And if your partner flatters you and wants you, your penis will respond positively, even when you do not think you are in the mood.

In my more than thirty years of practicing urology, I have observed a definite correlation between how men behave sexually and how they behave in general. Those with a negative penis image tend to have a poor self-image overall, while men with a positive penis image tend to see themselves in a positive light. For the most part, we behave in the bedroom much the way we behave in the living room, boardroom, factory, gym, or car.

In my practice, I have met innumerable penis personalities. I describe a few of these below. Any man might exhibit several of them or may shift from one to another. And these traits might apply equally to women and their vaginas.

The link between self-image and sexual identity is a critical point from which much of sexual weakness or sexual power stems. In order to better understand this correlation, think about your penis personality. Decide which traits you want to adopt and which you may need to reject. You may even have fun categorizing your friends' penis personalities. A willingness to examine yourself with the honest intent of improving who you are both as a person and as a sexual being will go a long way to enhancing your penis power.

The samples below offer just a few of the myriad personalities.

Positive Penis Personalities

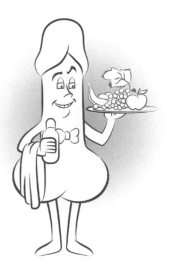

The Purposeful Penis Personality

The Purposeful Penis Personality approaches sex with his partner's satisfaction as his highest priority, learning the nuanced intricacies of her desires and applying his experience and skills to the fulfillment of those desires. He is thorough in his self-education, and his knowledge is always balanced by an educated sensitivity.

The Perceptive Penis Personality

The Perceptive Penis Personality empathizes with his partner, responding generously to his partner's needs and intuitively picking up on unexpressed moods and desires. It is as if his penis were a submarine periscope poking its head·above the surface into the light, always striving to make the best possible decisions.

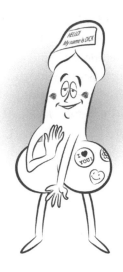

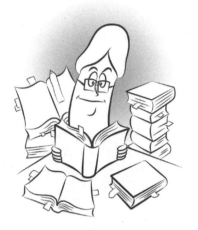

The Pensive Penis Personality

The Pensive Penis is intelligent, well informed, and clear thinking, probing for fresh ways to bring pleasure to his lover. There is a caveat. If he gets *too* calculating, he can miss out on a lot of fun.

The Passionate Penis Personality

He's Rhett Butler and Prince Charming, George Clooney and Brad Pitt, a lover's lover with boundless enthusiasm for life. Emotional, ardent, and lusty, he likes grand gestures and noble statements. He sends bouquets, dances cheek to cheek, remembers birthdays and anniversaries, and if he forgets, he will make up for his error magnificently. He is likely to have a clever nickname for his penis, which he regards as a staunch friend and trusted ally in the service of *l'amour*. Lovers find him irresistible because he is as sensitive as he is strong.

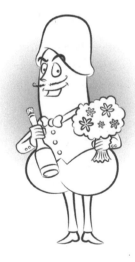

The Psychedelic Penis Personality

The Psychedelic Penis Personality is wild and experimental, and with him, the sexual experience is a vibrant swirl of colors, sounds, and emotional excitement. He takes sex *beyond* reality by adding new dimensions to old habits while maintaining the respect and sensitivity of a sane lover. He does not rely on drugs or illicit substances.

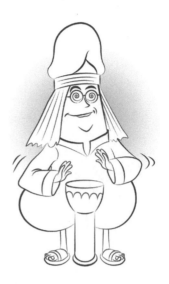

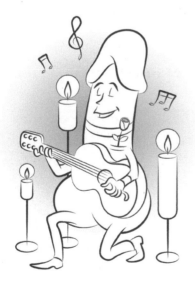

The Poetic Penis Personality

The Poetic Penis Personality speaks a language of love filled with deep thought, feeling, and life experience and makes every encounter a romantic tour de force. He makes love like a dancer, with poetry and precision in his every movement.

The Prodigious Penis Personality

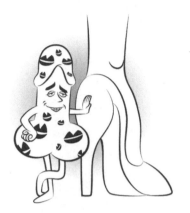

The Prodigious Penis Personality thinks and acts as if he is prodigiously large. He has a bustling libido and an abundant heart and a generous soul. He gives of himself freely and is ready for sex at any time and in any place. He has what I call penis largesse, extracting maximum pleasure from any situation. Women are drawn to him, sometimes for reasons they cannot explain.

These sample positive penis personalities represent those who have characteristics embodied in the *superpotent man*. Now let us look at a few sources of penis weakness.

Negative Penis Personalities

The Procrastinating Penis Personality

Why have sex here and now when you can put it off until tomorrow? That is what the Procrastinating Penis thinks. It is never the right time, place, or partner. The procrastinator is not lazy; he is so terrified of penis failure that he cannot bring himself to face the challenge.

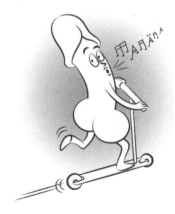

The Pompous Penis Personality

The Pompous Penis Personality is the locker-room braggart who spins crude tales about his conquests and his prodigious feats. This arrogant, self-important individual misrepresents himself to his partners. He promises a night of bliss but often falls short of his boastful arrogance. Be cautious with your arrogance. You may be the only one left to listen to your own bravado.

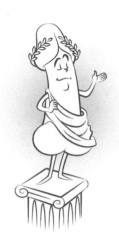

The Pipe-Dream Penis Personality

The Pipe-Dream Penis Personality lives in a world where he is a combination of Tommy Lee and Ron Jeremy and where flawless women lust for him and he satisfies their every desire. His mind is XXX-rated, but his penis is strictly Family Channel. I try to convince such men to be proud of what God has given them. If they accept the real sexual opportunities before them with gratitude, they do not have to live in a fantasy world.

The Pious Penis Personality

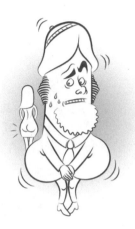

The Pious Penis Personality could be a minister, priest, rabbi, mullah, or even a devout layman trying to conform to scripture. Men who abstain from sex because of religious beliefs tend to be torn by conflict. Physiologically, these men have the same needs as everyone else, but many pious men manage to maintain vows while exhibiting joy and tolerance for those with more liberal attitudes. These men deserve and receive my respect. But the pious hypocrite who cavorts with hookers or molests children while threatening "sinners" with fire and damnation deserves neither respect nor pity.

The Pedestrian Penis Personality

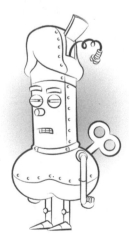

The Pedestrian Penis Personality is unimaginative, mechanical, and without spontaneity, the sexual equivalent of an automatic camera. I try, usually in vain, to get these guys to loosen up before they find themselves sexually dried up and alone.

The Pampered Penis Personality

The Pampered Penis Personality feels entitled to special treatment. You expect his penis to stand up and sing "Do things for me, buy things for me, cater to my every whim." The penis *should* be the center of attention, but demanding to be pampered without offering reciprocation or gratitude is not a sign of positive penis power—it is a sign of insecure neediness.

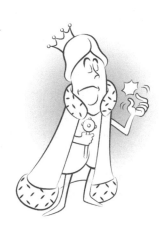

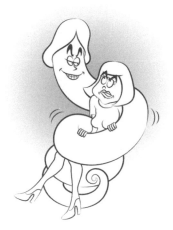

The Possessive Penis Personality

The Possessive Penis Personality does not want a lover; he wants an emotional and physical slave. Making some demands and insisting on fidelity are not signs of weakness, but this type wants to dominate and control his partner's life and every aspect of her sexuality to an unhealthy degree.

The personalities discussed in this chapter are universal and are a wonderful point of departure for discussions between partners. I urge all readers to take the necessary time to reflect on which of these personality traits, both positive and negative, they and their partners might have. If you and your partner have some of these negative qualities and they are having a harmful effect on your relationship, talk about these openly. Be honest. Recognize areas in your personality that may need adjustment, and help your partner to acknowledge whatever issues she may have. The future of your personal and sexual happiness rests on these fundamental psychological issues. To become a man of true penis power, you must have the courage and strength to change what is not working and create a path of change that leads to *superpotency*.

Chapter 14

What Is a Superpotent Man?

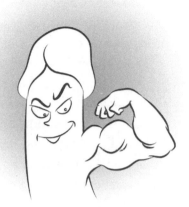

Having been privy to the intimate details of hundreds of thousands of patients' lives, as well as to those colleagues, friends, and family members who have taken advantage of my professional status and medical curiosity to discuss their sex lives, I have over the years developed a portrait of a special penis personality. This is the superpotent man.

Superpotency is a birthright and should be seen as a natural state of affairs. Every man can harness its power and reap its great rewards. As you read you might think, "I'll never be that kind of guy."

To that I say: "Nonsense!"

By the time you finish reading this book, you should be well on your way. Superpotency begins with thinking positively about yourself, your penis, and your sexuality.

Discovering Penis Power

You have seen those men who command attention, who turn heads when they enter a room. These men are magnetic. Strong and confident men view them with admiration and respect. Weaker men are awestruck or intimidated. Many are attracted to these individuals, both physically and mentally. You might call that certain something these men have presence or sex appeal or, simply, it. I call it penis power.

Penis power is not about status or money. It is especially not about penis size. Superpotent men are not necessarily hunks. There are handsome men with penis power and handsome men without it. The same is true for the guys some may find unattractive. The guy who has both looks and superpotency has a lot going for him. But between a handsome man without it and a homely man with it, the latter will attract more partners and lead a more satisfying life.

Take a look at celebrities who are considered sexy though not blessed with classic good looks. French actor Gérard Depardieu and American actor Owen Wilson both have doughy faces and oversized noses, yet there is no denying their sex appeal. I do not know either, but I would be willing to wager they possess abundant penis power, and not just because of their fame.

How about Jack Nicholson? He's balding and potbellied and still has something both women *and* men find irresistible. Several decades ago the film producer Carlo Ponti, a small, bald, ordinary-looking man, married gorgeous, talented, voluptuous, sexy Sophia Loren, the most desired woman in the world. And she *stayed* married to him.

On the flip side, I've seen many gorgeous hunks who satisfy every aesthetic criterion but arouse no attention, like the incredible physical specimen of a man who one day walked into my office for an appointment. He was a professional athlete with a body of solid muscle and a face worthy of the cover of *GQ*. I assumed he had women falling at his feet, so I teased the women in my office by asking who wanted to meet him. There were no takers.

"It's all on the outside," one of them explained when I expressed surprise at their disinterest. "He just doesn't have *it*."

Superpotency is not about looks. However, any man who desires penis power will take responsibility for his physical appearance by maintaining a healthy diet and exercise regimen. And men who develop the self-confidence and strength that are the foundation of penis power find that they look much better in the mind's eye.

Superpotency is not about wealth or social position. Superpotent men tend to be relatively successful because their personal qualities foster achievement. I cannot deny the fact that many people are attracted to rich and powerful men just because they are rich and powerful, but the appeal of wealth and status is superficial and does not qualify a man as superpotent. Once the Bentley is parked in its Beverly Hills garage and the $3,000 suit is in the closet, the rich man might be far less potent than the struggling artist in his garret or the assembly-line worker in his tract home. The only abundance that counts is an *attitude* of abundance—self-confidence in oneself and one's sexuality.

My patients and acquaintances are some of the richest and most influential people in the world, and many have true penis power, but a far greater number who are powerful in the office are plagued by penis weakness.

At the same time, I know men who lead humble lives yet are superpotent. Penis power emanates from the heart and soul of a man, and, in a word, it is priceless.

The Character of the Superpotent Man

What follows are the primary characteristics of superpotent men, characteristics within the reach of every man. As you read, ask yourself to what extent you possess these traits, and if you lack in a particular area, make it a personal goal to develop those traits as part of your efforts to maximize your penis power.

The Superpotent Man Exudes Self-Confidence

Superpotent men know who they are emotionally and spiritually. They feel good about themselves and their place in the world. They have a contentment but do not rest on their laurels. They are curious about life and always explore new opportunities with zeal. They thrive on new challenges and adventures.

The Superpotent Man Expresses His Full Potential

I often ask men, "What have you never done but want to do?" Super-potent men might mention a trip they have not yet taken or an ambitious task like "writing that novel." But they answer as if they know it will get done in time. Superpotent men do not live with regret.

A colleague of mine, a fellow of enormous penis power, captured this attitude best when we were on a trip together. As we were riding up a ski lift, I asked him if there was anything he had never done and wanted to do. The air was crisp, the sky crystal blue. My friend surveyed the glorious scene, reflected in silence, and finally said, "There are some things I'd still like to do. But if I were to die today, I would have no regrets." Superpotent men succeed because they exercise their full potential at every moment in their lives.

The Superpotent Man Is a Winner

The superpotent man not only is hardworking and passionate, but he also puts his heart and soul into all pursuits. Men with penis power naturally like competition, but their self-worth does not hinge on coming in first every time. Superpotent men enjoy the sheer exhilaration of working to achieve a goal. To these men, what truly matters is that they always try their best. When things go wrong, superpotent men bounce back quickly, using setbacks as motivation to forge ahead with even greater confidence. They reflect the emotional and psychological poise that any hardworking and determined individual can achieve.

The Superpotent Man Is Courageous

When the going gets tough, you want the superpotent man on your side. He thrives under pressure. He keeps his cool and takes charge in a crisis. Whether or not he is in a position of authority in the classic sense is unimportant. He adopts the attitude of a leader. He knows how to convert fear and tension into motivation and effective action. Super-potent men have the courage to face difficult challenges and the confidence to assume responsibility even when others are in charge.

The Superpotent Man Is Happy

If there were a motto for superpotency, it would probably be "Enjoy life to the fullest and the rest will follow." Superpotent men take advantage of the present moment, extracting positive aspects from every situation. Penis power and a good sense of humor go hand in hand. You don't have to be as funny as Chris Rock or Jim Carrey, but the twinkle in your eye should say, "I do not take myself *or* my life too seriously." You might be quiet and reserved or outgoing and extroverted, but fear, anxiety, and nervousness do not diminish your happiness. Superpotent men laugh just as exuberantly at their own foibles as they do at a good joke.

If life throws a tragedy at you, being sad and vulnerable is appropriate, of course, but superpotent men do not feel like victims. Learning how to handle the ups and downs of life is a crucial part of developing a healthy connection between your mind, sexuality, and penis.

The Superpotent Man Is Well Rounded

Superpotent men approach every activity with enthusiasm and appreciation. They usually have a wide range of interests, hobbies, and pursuits, and they love to learn. Becoming superpotent does not mean becoming involved in countless meaningless activities but being continuously interested in expanding your personality and knowledge.

The Superpotent Man Has Quality Relationships

Superpotent men work hard to have quality relationships in both their business and personal lives. A psychiatrist friend once told me that strong, successful men know that they *need* other people and understand they cannot achieve their goals alone. Superpotent men treat people with respect and, therefore, command the same from others. Their charm and ease emanates from their sensitivity to others' feelings.

The Superpotent Man and Sex

All the qualities described above are readily attainable if you are willing to adjust your beliefs and attitudes. If you have the courage to recognize areas in your life that need work and the strength to make changes, you will undoubtedly see huge improvements in your self-image, your interpersonal relationships, and every other area of your life. But let us look specifically at attitudes and behaviors of the superpotent man as they pertain to sex.

If you desire to become not only a great person but also a great lover, you must be willing to confront yourself and address the aspects of your personality that may be holding you back from emotional and sexual happiness. If you and your partner are having relationship problems because of personality or behavioral habits, having an open and honest discussion about the real issues involved is vital. Using this book as a guide is a great way to break the ice.

The Superpotent Man Has a Symbiotic Relationship with His Penis

Your penis is an integral part of your physical and emotional self. In a certain sense, your penis is your most vital organ. Of course, if your heart, lungs, and kidneys do not function properly you die, and this is not true of the penis. But your penis expresses your spirit and individuality.

The superpotent man loves his penis. He respects it. He treats it well.

Let me distinguish the man of penis power from those who *seem* to be. The superpotent man is not obsessed with or dominated by his penis. Men with penis power seldom *seem* penis oriented; rather, the superpotent man carries his penis with pride and with dignity, with nothing to prove and nothing to hide.

As an experienced urologist, I can assure you that the penis of a superpotent man has no special attributes that separate it from the penises of the rest of the species. The differences are all in the mind.

The Superpotent Man Has a High Level of Penis Awareness

He who understands his penis knows himself. Make an effort to learn about the anatomy and physiology of your penis, its likes and dislikes, quirks and foibles. Ultimately, your mind and your penis are controlled by the same axis. When you are tired or upset, your penis will behave that way, too. If you are angry, your penis will express that anger. If you adore your partner, your penis will show it.

Penis awareness creates harmonious functioning between your mind and your penis. The superpotent penis will do what its owner expects it to do. Like a trustworthy business partner, your penis is far less likely to disappoint you or come up with unpleasant surprises if you develop a healthy relationship with it.

The Superpotent Man Has an Extremely Satisfying Sex Life

The superpotent man does not measure his sexual self-worth by performance. Rather, he has a positive penis attitude. This is true for a single man with a variety of sex partners or a monogamous man with one partner for life. This is true whether the superpotent man is young and handsome or aging and ordinary.

Penis power is not about performing Olympian sexual feats. Superpotent men do not break records for frequency of intercourse, the number of orgasms their partners have, or the number of times they can achieve an erection in a night. If these were the criteria for penis power, pornographic film stars would be the epitome of penis power. They get erect on command and ejaculate whenever the director orders it. But I have treated many male pornographic film stars, and I would not categorize a single one as a superpotent man. They represent an inflated, overeroticized concept of male sexual power that has no relation to true penis power.

To be a superpotent man, you must view sex as an intimate pleasure, not a sporting event or show business. You are not there to prove anything or to perform for anyone. What should matter is that you use your penis as often and in such a manner as is most satisfying to both you and your partner. What you should care about is that, when you call upon your penis, it functions according to your personal standards. That is not to say that the penis of a superpotent man always performs to maximum capacity, but because his penis functions in harmony with the rest of his mind and body, its success rate is much higher than the penises of most men. When the man of penis power is let down by his penis, he takes it in stride and knows that *such occurrences happen to all men* and are to be expected from time to time. What others see as a problem, the man of penis power might see as a joke or an opportunity to face another penis challenge. The superpotent man learns from experience and moves ahead to the next sexual opportunity without hesitation or apprehension.

The Superpotent Man Enjoys Giving and Receiving Pleasure

Not only does the superpotent man have sex often; he also savors each experience. Be passionate and intense during sex. Be frivolous, whimsical, and funny if the occasion calls for it. It is okay to laugh during sex, even at yourself. The superpotent man enjoys spontaneity and unpredictability and appreciates imaginative partners.

The Superpotent Man Enjoys Variety

Most men of penis power thrive on variety, which may mean frequent encounters with an assortment of partners, or it may mean a wide spectrum of adventures with one partner. This riddle epitomizes the attitude:

What is the difference between sex and wrestling?
Answer: In wrestling, some holds are barred.

Superpotent men are not womanizers or "players"; even those who move from bed to bed pursue their pleasure responsibly. Penis power, as with all types of power, carries with it moral obligations. A superpotent man never exploits or abuses but applies his penis power with generosity and sensitivity. Superpotent men are not promiscuous and do not pursue pleasure at the expense of a balanced life or at the cost of hurting others. The goal is mutual enjoyment, not sexual conquest.

Like an experienced commuter who does not risk his life by running wildly down the track to catch a train because he knows another will come shortly, superpotent men know that tomorrow is another day, and they do not take foolish risks. They are aware of the ramifications of their actions. As a urologist who has watched patients waste away and die of HIV/AIDS, I urge you to educate yourself about sexually transmitted diseases and to exercise your penis power prudently. You do not need to be paranoid, but you must know the facts. (See more in chapter 10.)

The Superpotent Man Is at Ease with His Sexuality

The superpotent man loves sex and thinks about it often. And like other men of genuine talent and ability, the man of penis power lets his good performances speak for themselves.

Despite the rhetoric of extremists, most people understand that an appreciation of the human form is healthy, and that the body is designed to arouse sexual interest. Our desire to attract inspires us to dress well, to fuss with our hair, to accentuate the positives in our physiques. The man of penis power appreciates the human form in all its shapes and sizes: the shape of a leg, the curve of a hip, and the swelling arc of a full bosom or buttock. This natural urge is all part of nature's plan for keeping the species alive, and the superpotent man acknowledges, celebrates, and enjoys it.

Let me make an important point: on some level, superpotent men view their partners as sex objects, but they do not view them as mere sex objects.

They may not admit it, but deep in the corners of their psyche, all men see their partners as the means to a definitive sexual end, and women see men as sex objects as well. But superpotent men appreciate all dimensions of their lovers. While he loves sex, loves to chase after sexual opportunities, and will pursue a liaison with persistence, he understands the fine line in the delicate dance of sex and always behaves with sensitivity, awareness, and integrity. He respects boundaries and never ever forces or ignores the partner who says no!

As a surgeon, I often say you can teach a gorilla how to do an appendectomy, but you cannot teach a gorilla when to do one. That takes *judgment*, and in sexual behavior, as in surgery, judgment separates the superpotent men from the boys.

The Superpotent Man Gives Openly and without Reservation

Superpotent men understand the importance of open, honest communication. You should care about your partner's sexual pleasure, not for the sake of macho pride or because you are a self-sacrificing saint. You should care because you value your partner's satisfaction and know that the more you give, the more you will receive in return. When a partner tells the superpotent man she likes or dislikes what he is doing, he does his best to accommodate her preferences, sometimes paying attention to subtle clues. If you ask your partner if what you are doing is good or bad, you'll be a man of penis power. Talking about sex while it is happening is not only a huge turnon to many, it is also a guaranteed way to find out how to satisfy your partner. The same goes for unreservedly expressing your own needs and desires.

The Superpotent Man Does Not Have Performance Anxiety

Perhaps the most salient distinction between men with penis power and men with penis weakness is the presence or absence of performance anxiety. Several studies have been done in which sex partners are observed in aroused states, usually brought on by the viewing of erotic videos.[1]

The men who stated at the beginning of the studies that they performed in a satisfactory manner showed a marked increase in arousal after viewing the erotic films in sharp contrast with the men who had admitted some degree of sexual dysfunction. That second group had a marked *decrease* in arousal after watching the movies. Why? Because as their partners became more responsive, they began to concentrate on performance anxieties they associated with sex. The more confident men focused on the erotic cues of their aroused partners and got even more turned on.

Men of penis weakness have a negative feedback loop. A sexual proposition elicits a negative expectation that leads to self-consciousness that leads to an inability to perceive a partner's cues, which leads to decreased arousal. This path confirms negative expectations, increasing performance anxiety and preventing adequate performance. All of this leads to future avoidance of sex and future failure.

In sharp contrast, men of penis power develop a positive feedback loop that starts with an aroused partner or an invitation to sex. This immediately registers a positive expectation and is followed by an accurate assessment of the sexual demand and a direct focus on meeting that demand. Men of penis power focus on the wonderful experience they are about to share, and this automatically leads to greater penis arousal, which loops around to a heightened attention to sexual cues. A mutually satisfying sexual experience and an increase in confidence result.

To become a man of penis power, you must become a master of the positive sexual feedback loop.

The Superpotent Man Knows How to Handle Stress

Superpotent men do not succumb to the debilitation of anxiety or depression.

Nothing is more debilitating to sexual satisfaction than anxiety and depression. Although depression is known to diminish sexual desire and responsiveness, this result is not inevitable. Even a superpotent man is vulnerable to the worries and fears that afflict all people at one time or another and to occasional situational depression. But, if you have faith in yourself, develop a healthy method for dealing with your emotions, and learn how to extract the positive elements from every experience, you will climb out of depressions quickly and convert your worries into effective action.

To become a man of penis power, you must develop the capacity to prevent negative emotions from impeding your ability to achieve an erection. You cannot let the stress of your outside life intrude into the bedroom.

Penis Power Is Defined by Who You Are and How You Control Your Life

You should now have a clear understanding of the chief characteristics of superpotent men, though superpotent men are not shaped by the same cookie cutter. They share the majority of these important behavioral and attitudinal patterns but also exhibit a tremendous range of variation. They are tall and short, plain and handsome, young and old, rich and poor. Their penises are big, small, and average. They have sex all the time, frequently, or only occasionally. They are bold and aggressive or shy and self-effacing. They like blondes, brunettes, or redheads and partners who are tall, short, buxom, or slim. During sex they prefer the missionary position, sitting up, the canine way, their partner on top—or all of the above. They like sex in the morning, at night, in the afternoon, or at all times of day.

Discovering your penis power does not happen by imitating or by living up to a hypothetical standard. Penis power comes from examining those aspects of your personality, relationships, and self-image that you want to improve and then making needed changes. Penis power is about self-understanding and self-expression. Most of all, it is about realizing your full potential. Your way of expressing penis power is as good as anyone else's way. What's important is harnessing that power and using it to extract the most pleasure from your entire life.

Superpotency is normal and natural and within your reach. You will be surprised at how easy it is to achieve. Self-doubt, and the penis weakness it creates, is a *temporary* sickness. I have seen men become superpotent after learning a few facts and listening to a simple pep talk. They readjust their attitudes about themselves and their penises, adopting positive personality traits and rejecting the negative traits that were holding them back. After that, they're off and running with nearly immediate great results. Others have to work at it for some time or must use the specific tips found in this book to change their sexual behavior, increase their penis power, and prove to themselves and their partners that they are capable of being superpotent.

Chapter 15

How to Become a Superpotent Man

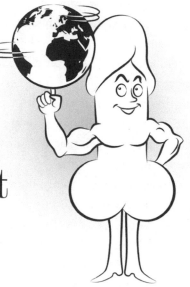

Y*ou* can be a superpotent man. Every man can. This chapter offers practical steps you can take to maximize your penis power. I must emphasize that the most important steps you can take are to work hard to maintain physical fitness and to cultivate a happy, upbeat attitude toward life as a whole. Superpotency is nothing more than expressing your life force and energy through the power of your penis and your sexuality. Develop the positive qualities of a superpotent man (see chapter 14). If you emulate these and shape your behavior and attitude accordingly, increasing your penis power will be easy and effective.

Educate Yourself

I am constantly amazed by men's ignorance about sexuality in general and women in particular. I have known men with highly sophisticated minds, wide-ranging experience, and excellent educations who do not know a clitoris from a cuticle, and not because they are uninterested in sex. On the contrary, they are *very* interested but complain that they cannot "figure women out." The problem comes from their being overly interested in their own satisfaction and not interested enough in their partners'.

Part of becoming superpotent involves caring a great deal about satisfying your partner's needs and desires, not just out of generosity and a belief in equality but also out of pure *self-interest*. I am not certain about the rest of life, but in sex you really do reap what you sow. Satisfy your lover, and she will react by finding ways to please you in a manner you never thought possible.

We know that women are different from men, but a heterosexual man of penis power should understand *exactly how* women are different. Many books are devoted entirely to women's sexuality—and all men should be experts. But I would like to single out one point that many men do not fully appreciate. For physiological reasons, women generally take longer than men to get aroused. As one of my patients observed, "Women are like radio tubes—it takes them time to warm up. Men are like transistors—solid-state and turned on instantly." Women often complain that men denigrate foreplay, and men complain that women want to fool around too much before "getting down to business."

Each partner must learn to accommodate the other. If a man is sometimes so turned on that he has no time for the niceties of foreplay, his partner should try to understand this particularly urgent expression of passion. All men, regardless of their passionate urges, must learn to appreciate a partner's desire for the subtle and sensual pleasures of foreplay and learn to satisfy this need with patience and generosity. Technically, foreplay is necessary to lubricate a woman's vagina, and if you are impatient, you might be missing out on some of life's sweetest pleasures and depriving yourself of the great satisfaction that comes from giving pleasure to your partner.

Even more important than understanding women's sexuality in general is learning about your specific partner's sexuality. Women have a vast range of likes and dislikes. Never assume that the partner you are with has the same sexual preferences as your past partners.

Honest and open communication is essential. Many men are uncomfortable talking about sex, even with long-term partners, but if you want to be a superpotent man, you must find out what most pleases your partner. A partner who is open and honest is one of the best allies a penis can have.

Equally important is a partner who is responsive to your needs. I'm amazed by how many men complain to me that their lovers do not do enough of this or do too much of that but never bother to discuss this dissatisfaction with them. Be up front about your preferences. Communicate without pressure, criticism, or ultimatums. If she is willing to make the effort, it will surely enhance your penis power. If she is not willing, you might be in a sexually incompatible relationship, or you might have to sort out some of the deeper reasons for her resistance. Unless your desires run to dangerous sex or your partner has personal limitations and boundaries, you deserve to have your wishes met; in turn, you also must be willing to meet your partner halfway.

A final word to those learning about sex: If you overanalyze it, you paralyze it. Do not overintellectualize. You can get so bogged down with facts and diagrams and psychological theories that you end up being even more self-conscious and inhibited than you were when you started.

Good Health Equals Good Penis Power

The general condition of your mind and body is reflected in the health of your penis power. Maintain a high level of well-being, both mentally and physically.

Get Fit and Stay Fit

A good exercise program is central to overall health and sexual fitness. The muscles of your arms, legs, back, and abdomen are all involved in making love. If they become flabby, your penis also risks becoming flabby. Build up your muscular strength with weights, push-ups, sit-ups, yoga, or whatever exercise you prefer. You need not be "ripped" or sculpted like a Greek god, but muscular strength and flexibility are important.

Commit to Cardiovascular Fitness

I recommend a vigorous half hour of aerobic exercises four or five times a week for developing and maintaining cardiovascular fitness. Physical inactivity leads to deterioration of your body as a whole and can also lead to deterioration of your penis power. If you start wheezing or gasping for breath while making love, your penis will get the message that you need to rest, and it will.

Pay Attention to What You Eat

A diet low in saturated fat and high in fiber is most effective for maintaining penis power. Superpotency depends on clean arteries to support blood flow for keeping an erection. Ingesting saturated fats and bad cholesterol gums up the works. While wining and dining can be romantic, the romance withers if you wind up bloated or constipated. Too much alcohol (or any intoxicant) might increase your desire but will surely diminish your penis power. In addition, a superpotent man should be concerned with maintaining good prostate health. Reliable evidence supports a low-fat, high-fiber, and high-protein diet in addition to regular exercise as part of a good overall regimen to keep your prostate healthy.

Maintain Weight Control

Let's face it—operating smoothly and vigorously in bed is a lot easier if you are not carrying a twenty-pound belt of blubber around your waist. Being overweight brings health risks, and for most, a lean physique is much more attractive. Even more important than how other people see you is *your* perception of your body. Maintaining a healthy body weight encourages self-confidence. In addition, if you are overweight and looking down at your penis from above a big belly, you might start thinking of your penis as small because layers of fat obscure so much of it and in turn, you will *think* small about your penis power.

Men who are comfortable with their bodies have a higher likelihood for superpotency, but these men are not necessarily hunks. Some good-looking, well-built men are so insecure and vain that if they do not see

Brad Pitt when they look in the mirror, they hate their bodies, and ultimately their self-esteem suffers. Every man is capable of realizing his personal body image goals. To start, set your own standards of health and fitness and maintain a regular routine.

Do Not Hold Your Penis Power Hostage to the Youth Cult Perpetuated by the Media

Those images of sleek, muscular bodies with gorgeous women at their sides promoting everything from deodorant to pickup trucks are detrimental to superpotency. Who could possibly live up to those standards? Avoid comparing yourself to other men, especially those airbrushed images.

Get Plenty of Rest

Superpotent men live balanced lives. They are energetic, busy, and productive, but they are not obsessive about work. In my experience, many workaholics drown themselves in work to make up for some deep feeling of inadequacy, and in turn, they often jeopardize good relationships. Superpotent men are usually just as productive and work just as hard, but they also know when and how to relax. Their capacity for fun is as big as their capacity for work. They have that seemingly uncanny ability to compartmentalize their lives.

Maintain Good Mental Health

Penis power also requires sound mental health. Stress will weaken you physically, interfere with the biochemical action needed to produce erections, and possibly lower your self-image to the point where you doubt your manhood. Numerous studies have shown that people who undergo major traumas, such as the loss of a loved one or a serious accident, are much more likely to experience serious illness. I can add unequivocally that they are also more likely to exhibit penis weakness. I have seen many patients suffering from posttraumatic stress disorder, and their penises often behave just like the men themselves: confused, frightened, and helpless. My superpotent patients deal with even serious trauma in a healthy, effective way. When the crisis resolves, they put it behind them, and their stressful encounter fades quickly from their minds. If you do not learn to deal with life's difficulties in a positive way, traumas large and small will pollute all aspects of your life.

Penis Power Exercises

Sex is the best way to develop penis power! Just like in a sports stadium or concert hall, practice makes perfect in bed. The more you use your penis and the more you learn about using it, the more control you will gain over its functioning. Making love is a great form of exercise for your whole body. Vigorous sex increases the volume of oxygen in your lungs, quickens your heart rate, and raises your effective circulating blood volume, all of which benefit your general health. Sex can also help you moderate potentially dangerous habits. When you are sexually satisfied, you feel so good about yourself that you are less likely to abuse drugs, alcohol, or junk food. Finally, sex is a great antidote for stress (if not the greatest!).

There is no sense in exercising the penis itself because, physically speaking, it is a passive organ, with no muscles. However, you can exercise other body parts that serve the penis during sex. Push-ups or weight exercises that use the same basic motion of pushing and pulling with the upper arms and chest muscles are suggested. To the extent that you support your body with your arms while making love, this conditioning will help prevent fatigue, so that your penis will not be thinking, "Hurry up and get it over with!" Squats, knee bends, or other exercises for the upper legs, as well as exercises that strengthen the abdominal muscles, will all increase penis power, helping to support you during various sexual positions.

Maybe Elvis Was on to Something: Pelvic Control

If you have control of your pelvis, your penis will function more creatively and dynamically. Sit-ups, crunches, leg raises, and similar exercises will strengthen the muscles of the abdomen and lower back. More to the point, I advise working on the flexibility of the pelvic region itself.

Lucien Martin, a chiropractor in Santa Monica, California, created a series of exercises to strengthen the muscles of the lower back and abdomen for patients with back problems. To his surprise, his patients reported dramatic improvements in their sex lives. According to Dr. Martin, the exercises strengthen the muscles and ligaments of the pelvis, lower back, and abdomen, and they seem to improve nerve sensitivity in that area.

Dr. Martin's instructions for his pelvic control technique are as follows:

> Lie on your back on the floor or on a very firm bed, arms at your sides. Place a tightly rolled towel of three to four inches in diameter under your neck, not your head. Place a thick pillow under your knees so that your lower back rests flat on the floor.

> Without lifting your lower back off the floor, pull your pubic bone toward your chest. Do not suck in your stomach. The idea is to lift the pelvis by *squeezing* the abdominals like an accordion, not to pull them inward.

> Lock the pelvis in the compressed position for a second and then relax. Repeat the same pattern again and again.

> To make sure you are doing it correctly, press your lower abdominal muscles with the fingers of both hands as you squeeze. You should feel those core muscles contract. Another way to test yourself is to press the abdominal muscles while slightly raising your head and legs. You should feel the compression of the muscles used.

> Proper breathing is important. Keep your throat and mouth relaxed. As you squeeze, let the motion of your pelvis expel air from your lungs. Do not breathe out

forcefully, and do not hold your breath. Exhale smoothly as you contract your abdominals, and inhale smoothly as you relax.

The exercise should be brief and vigorous. Hold each contraction for about a second and continue the repetitions for two to three minutes.

Once you gain good control, you can set a goal of one hundred repetitions per day.

One note of caution: if you have acute lower back problems, do not undertake this exercise without first consulting your orthopedist.

The Harder They Come: Controlling Your Timing

Superpotency is about not only getting an erection at the right time but also controlling the timing of your orgasm, and as discussed in chapter 4, problems with ejaculation usually come in two categories: too fast or too slow.

A too-slow ejaculation, or retarded ejaculation, can be caused by such medical factors as spinal cord injury or diabetes, as well as by substance abuse or the side effects of certain medications. In rare instances, the problem is so extreme that a man may be unable to ejaculate at all. Obviously, this requires the attention of a urologist. In other cases, the problem is psychological. Some men can masturbate to climax *and* even have nocturnal emissions (spontaneous ejaculation at night), but cannot ejaculate in a vagina or with their partners. This is usually rooted in self-doubt, repressed trauma, fear of pregnancy, or anxiety and can best be dealt with by psychological counseling.

The normal aging process is by far the most common reason for retarded ejaculation, but men who develop problems controlling their ejaculate might come to view this as a positive development because sex lasts longer, and both partners are more satisfied. This can be problematic, especially in an older couple exhausting themselves by pumping away to induce an orgasm while the vagina becomes irritated. For an older couple, patience and lubrication will usually solve the problem. I suggest you vary your positions and avoid particularly strenuous sexual activities. Do not hesitate to rest when you need to. Experiment with oils and lotions—lubrication might increase sensitivity enough to facilitate orgasm.

The more troubling problem is premature ejaculation. As discussed in chapter 4, some variation exists in the way the medical community defines premature ejaculation. Some sex therapists classify it as the inability to delay ejaculation for at least five minutes. Others define it as the inability to delay ejaculation long enough to satisfy your partner in at least half of your sexual encounters. That perspective recognizes that it is normal for the time of ejaculation to vary and to sometimes fall short of the ideal.

Coming up with a universal definition is impossible because so much variation occurs among individuals. It comes down to individual judgment: Do you and your partner feel that you reach orgasm too quickly? If so, there are many practical steps you can take.

The most common cause of premature ejaculation is sexual inactivity. When the seminal vesicles are filled to capacity, it takes very little stimulation to start the ejaculatory reflex because the fluid simply has to be released. This is why every man experiences quick ejaculation on occasion and why it happens most often to younger men who produce a much larger *volume* of seminal fluid. The ejaculatory reflex is volume related.

However, infrequent sex is not the only cause. When premature ejaculation becomes chronic, it is usually because of patterns rooted in early experience. For many young men, initial sexual encounters are characterized not only by anxiety and fear but also by time pressure. Teenagers who masturbate under their sheets can become self-conscious to the point of paranoia. Their goal is not to *delay*, but to get it over with as quickly as possible before they are discovered.

Ultimately, these types of early experiences establish a *low threshold of excitement*. Most men who develop this low threshold become conditioned to ejaculate quickly. I have often treated young men who are so humiliated by premature ejaculation that they develop a strong sense of inadequacy and shy away from sex altogether. Whatever the initial cause, do not view early ejaculation as a personal failure. If it occasionally happens, a long lapse between orgasms or nervousness is probably the cause. Even if the problem is chronic, it is not a sign of permanent inadequacy or diminished manhood but simply a matter of bad habits that can be changed.

No matter where you start, you can vastly increase your ejaculatory control. Using the procedures described below, I have helped patients who reached orgasm in less than two minutes improve to where they could last more than half an hour after a few weeks or months of practice.

One point is important: if you are in an ongoing relationship, it is important to win the support of your partner. If early ejaculation continues for a long time, it can lead to resentment. Many women have told me that they sometimes feel that their men care only about their own needs. Some say they feel used. You must convince your partner that you are sincere about improving your staying power and would be grateful for your partner's patience and help. The goal is to delay ejaculation to a point that is most satisfying for *both* of you.

The "Taint" Exercises

The following exercise, similar to that developed by gynecologist Arnold Kegel for female patients with urinary incontinence, will help give you greater control of your ejaculations and also increase the intensity of your orgasms.

The muscles in the perineum (the taint)—the area between the scrotum and the anus—are involved in the ejaculatory process. If you were to put your finger in that area when you ejaculate, you would feel the contractions. If you placed a mirror between your legs, you would see the whole area contract like a flexing bicep. Anatomically, these muscles support the urinary sphincter and are the muscles you contract when you are forced to hold in your urine. Try it the next time you urinate: when you stop the flow, the muscles you contract are the very ones we are talking about. By strengthening the muscles of the perineum, you will pump more blood to this vital area, achieve greater ejaculatory control, and increase the intensity of your orgasms.

The idea is to contract and relax the muscles repeatedly, either while standing up or sitting down. Use your mind's eye to isolate the muscles surrounding the anal sphincter. Imagine that you have inserted a rectal thermometer and are trying to pull it up into your body, right up to your Adam's apple. Do not hunch and do not squeeze your buttocks together. The muscles involved are all internal. Squeeze them and hold that position for ten counts. Then relax and repeat the process several times.

As with any new exercise, at first the muscles will feel tired. Do not do it to exhaustion; increase the number of repetitions until you can comfortably do one hundred a day. Do these exercises consistently and in time you will notice the benefits. Once you notice improvement, continue to do the exercises to maintain the improvement and progress even further. You can do them anytime: while driving, walking, standing in line, watching television. When done correctly, they are unobtrusive. If someone can tell you're doing the exercise, you are doing it wrong.

Techniques for Delaying Ejaculation

The key to prolonging intercourse is to become so well tuned to your own body mechanisms that you can take action to hold off ejaculation *before* it is too late. Remember, ejaculation is a two-step process. As arousal increases, you eventually reach ejaculatory inevitability, the moment when you feel that you are going to climax and nothing you can do will stop it. Physiologically speaking, you are correct. Once that point is reached, the ejaculation reflex is set in motion, the muscles of the perineum forcefully contract, and the seminal fluid is already on its way out. To delay ejaculation, you must be aware enough to do something *before* the point of inevitability. The first step is to pay close attention to physical sensations as you approach ejaculation. That is the time to make adjustments. Some men distract themselves by thinking of baseball or work or anything nonsexual. Unfortunately, even if this does slow the process, it also separates you from the intimate connection and detracts from your full enjoyment. A more effective and enjoyable technique is to change the angle, speed, or depth of your thrust; this will shift the sensations away from the head of your penis, thereby delaying ejaculation. The secret is to pay attention to the sensitivities of your own body and make the appropriate adjustments.

You can make love slowly. You can move in a circular motion or enter only partway. You can also stop thrusting entirely, a great way to reduce arousal and prolong intercourse. When you feel you can resume thrusting without ejaculating immediately, resume slowly.

Another variable is to withdraw entirely. Sex therapists often use this start-and-stop method. When you feel yourself nearing inevitability, simply pull out and rest. This is the time for using your hands, lips, tongue, and any other body part that gives you pleasure. When you resume, intercourse will be that much more intense, and your total time of penetration will increase. Do not be afraid of losing your erection. You *might*, but so what? It will come back with the right stimulation.

Squeeze Me, Please Me

One of the best methods of delaying ejaculation is the squeeze technique. When you feel you are close to ejaculation, withdraw your penis and grip the head (the glans) at the juncture where it meets the shaft, holding your thumb on the upper surface and your first and second fingers underneath. On the head, squeeze forcefully. This will delay the urge to ejaculate. The amount of pressure needed varies among men, but do not be afraid to squeeze hard. When the urge is gone, wait a moment or two before resuming intercourse. You may partially lose your erection after the squeeze, but that is *usually* not a problem. If it happens, remain relaxed, and your full erection will return shortly, especially if your penis has fresh stimulation.

Some of my patients say they prefer to have their partner do the squeezing, but I have found it more reliable for the patient to do it himself since familiarity helps him know when and exactly how firmly to squeeze. This technique is also used by my colleagues in sex therapy *without intercourse* as a method of systematically reconditioning men with long histories of premature ejaculation. In this process, the woman stimulates the man as if masturbating him but stops and squeezes when he signals that he is about to ejaculate. You are welcome to try this—there is nothing like on-the-job training.

The Valsalva Maneuver

The Valsalva maneuver involves holding your breath and bearing down with your abdominal muscles as if you were going to relieve stuffed bowels. You obviously squeeze your anal sphincter at the same time, so that you do not *actually* move your bowels. This creates a marked increase in intra-abdominal pressure and will delay the ejaculatory mechanism. As with the squeeze technique, timing is critical. If you do it too soon, it will not help. If you wait too long, you might reach the point of no return. Some men continue thrusting while doing the Valsalva maneuver, while others find it more comfortable to stop for a moment until they feel they can resume without exceeding the threshold of inevitability.

Following the techniques described above should extend your staying power significantly. Please bear in mind that no matter how much you improve your self-control, there will always be moments when you will ejaculate sooner than you would like. Don't apologize. If you ejaculate before your partner is satisfied, try other means besides intercourse to bring your partner to an orgasm. If you leave your partner frustrated, make up for it the next time. When you feel yourself slip into that zone where you lose control, do not resist the inevitable—just relax and enjoy it.

Eliminate Negativity and Self-Doubt

Self-doubt can wilt your penis power like frost on a rose petal, so eliminating self-doubt should be your priority in your quest for superpotency.

Of course you make mistakes. Of course you have weak spots and insecurities. We all do. A superpotent man faces his imperfections with honesty and humor and never lets anything obscure his basic and unconditional self-acceptance. Act like a winner in life, and you will be a winner in bed. Face the world with courage, and your penis will be courageous. Go through life with a smile on your face, and your penis will smile. Extract every drop of pleasure that life offers you, and your penis will make you doubly happy.

Do Not View Sex as a Performance

Stop thinking about sex as a stage production, an athletic event, or an exercise on which you are being graded, and you will eliminate performance anxiety. If you find yourself thinking about how you are going to perform when you are in bed, you are on the wrong track. Instead, visualize yourself enjoying every moment of the anticipated sexual encounter. Go into it expecting nothing from yourself other than to experience and give pleasure. Remove all standards of performance from your mind. Take the experience as it comes.

Your attitude toward your penis should be governed by the same positive reinforcement you would give to a child who is playing a soccer game or taking an exam: "I don't care if you win or lose. All that matters is that you give it your best shot." Ultimately, your capacity to relax and enjoy the intimacy and romance of sex is all that matters.

If your partner is too demanding, if her expectations are unrealistic, or if she compares you to other men, know that the problem is *hers*, not yours. Yes, you have a responsibility to try your best to satisfy your partner, but all you can do is give it your best effort, and if you have, you have no reason to feel guilty or ashamed.

Make Friends with Your Penis

Like any other part of your body, your penis is out in the world representing you. It reflects what you think of yourself and your life. Love your penis. Respect it, treat it well, take pride in it, and have faith in it. Your penis is your friend, and you should treat it accordingly.

If your penis has let you down and you have come to mistrust it, it is time to forgive and move on. Take responsibility for previous failures. Your penis is only an emissary that follows orders from your brain, and we all know better than to kill the messenger.

Take a good look at your penis in the mirror, and see it for the beautiful, whimsical organ that it is—court jester and sage rolled into one. Touch it, massage it with lotion, or sprinkle it with fragrance. Men shouldn't be ashamed to treat their genitals with the same special care with which they treat the rest of their bodies. Treat your penis with respect, and it will serve you with dignity.

A Final Word to Women

That last sentence can also be rephrased for women: treat his penis with respect, and it will serve *you* with dignity. While this chapter is directed to men, I sincerely hope women will use the information to help the men in their lives achieve their superpotency. Women who know how to attend to their men's penises have better relationships and better sex. If you take some of the time you spend trying to look attractive to men and use it to directly satisfy their sexual needs (both mentally and physically), you will attain far greater fulfillment.

Being penis oriented elevates your status because it enables you to have greater control and power in your relationship. Taking the time to understand what makes your man tick and learning to satisfy his penis needs does not make you subservient. Rather, by taking the initiative, you can establish a precedent that your man can be expected to follow *quid pro quo*.

More than thirty years of clinical experience have convinced me that an intelligent woman knows that one of the best ways to a man's heart and soul is through his penis.

A Final Word to Men

Penis power is not about size or the number of sexual conquests. It is not about blood vessels and nerves. Rather, penis power is about heightened self-awareness and an enthusiastic, conciliatory, and understandingly assertive attitude in life. Penis power is about admiring and respecting a body part that is never out of style, can never be overused, and will never wear out. It is about letting your penis read your mind and allowing your mind's voice to cry out, "My penis is *great*, and if it is great, *I am great*! It is Mr. Happy, and I am Mr. Happy!"

Penis power is a priceless luxury readily available to every man to be shared in every relationship throughout a lifetime of intimacy and compassion. Penis power is about communication and sensitivity between lovers, about sharing the mystique of man's most enigmatic body part with understanding and enthusiasm. Penis power is about emotional and sexual generosity. Penis power is about realizing that your penis is one of life's greatest gifts and that penis power is your own personal achievement. This power is to be shared wisely with your mate so that together you can soar to new heights of pleasure and intimacy.

As a penis doctor, I recommend that you use this book to develop communication skills with your penis. Whatever you do, *do not lose faith in your ability to improve your sexuality*.

I truly believe that a wise man would rather be a pauper and use his penis like a king than be a king who is incapable of exercising and sharing his right to penis power.

Acknowledgments

Special thanks to my dear wife, Hedva, without whom none of this would be possible. I am grateful to my daughter, Aurele Danoff, for her invaluable perspective and support. Thanks to my son, Doran A. Danoff, for his editorial assistance and insights in helping to create this book. And an extra-special thanks to my longtime friend and professional colleague Dr. Leo Gordon for his impeccable sense of literacy and for his professorial advice in helping to edit the final draft of this book.

And dare I forget to thank the women who have influenced my life—both through my practice and personal endeavors—for their unique perspective and wisdom. They have allowed me to express my ideas with a passion not otherwise possible.

Notes

Chapter 1

1. *Macbeth: A Tragedy*, ed. Samuel Johnson and George Steevens (London: Mathews and Leigh, 1807), act 2, sc. 3.

Chapter 3

1. Staff of the Institute for Sex Research, Indiana University, *Sexual Behavior in the Human Female* (Bloomington: Indiana University Press, 1953), 594.

Chapter 4

1. Anthony M. A. Smith et al., "Cannabis Use and Sexual Health," *Journal of Sexual Medicine* 7, no. 2 (February 2010): 787–793, doi:10.1111/j.1743-6109.2009.01453.x.

2. Anna Hodgekiss, "Smoking Cannabis Really *Does* Make People Lazy Because It Affects the Area of the Brain Responsible for Motivation," *Daily Mail*, July 1, 2013, http://www.dailymail.co.uk/health/article-2352695/Smoking-cannabis-really-DOES-make-people-lazy-affects-area-brain-responsible-motivation.html.

3. J. R. Kovac et al., "Effects of Cigarette Smoking on Erectile Dysfunction," *Andrologia* 47, no. 10 (December 2015): 1087–1092.

4. D. Rowland, J. Barada, and S. Bull, "Ratings of Factors Contributing to Overall Sexual Satisfaction in Men with and without Self-Reported Premature Ejaculation," *Journal of Sexual Medicine* 1 (2004): 58,094, cited in Chris G. McMahon, "Premature Ejaculation," *Indian Journal of Urology* 23, no. 2 (April–June 2007): 97–108, doi:10.4103/0970-1591.32056.

5. Omer Cakir, Brian Helfand, and Kevin McVary, "The Frequencies and Characteristics of Men Receiving Medical Intervention for Erectile Dysfunction: Analysis of 6.2 Million Patients," *Journal of Urology* 189, no. 4 (April 2013): 570, doi:10.1016/j.juro.2013.02.2747.

Chapter 5

1. National Cancer Institute Surveillance, Epidemiology, and End Results Program, "Cancer Stat Facts: Prostate Cancer," National Institutes of Health,

accessed February 10, 2017, http://seer.cancer.gov/statfacts/html/prost.
html.

2. "Company Profile," Intuitive Surgical, accessed February 3, 2017, http://
www.intuitivesurgical.com/company/profile.html.

3. Craig R. Ramsay, et al., "Ablative Therapy for People with Localised Prostate
Cancer: A Systematic Review and Economic Evaluation, *Health Technology
Assessment* 19, no. 49 (July 2015), doi:10.3310/hta19490.

Chapter 6

1. National Kidney and Urologic Diseases Information Clearinghouse, "Erectile
Dysfunction," National Institutes of Health, November 2015, http://www.
niddk.nih.gov/-/media/Files/Urologic-Diseases/Erectile_Dysfunction_Sec-
tion_508.pdf.

2. Hunter Wessells et al., "Erectile Dysfunction and Peyronie's Disease" in
Urologic Diseases in America, ed. Mark S. Litwin and Christopher S. Saigal
(Washington, DC: Government Printing Office, 2007), chap. 15.

3. C. C. Carson et al., "The Efficacy of Sildenafil Citrate (Viagra) in Clinical Pop-
ulations: An Update," *Urology* 60, no. 2, suppl. 2 (September 2002): 12–27.

4. Ibid.

5. "Muse," Drugs.com, last modified December 2015, http://www.drugs.com/
pro/muse.html.

Chapter 7

1. Warren G. Bennis, *An Invented Life: Reflections on Leadership and Change* (New
York: Basic Books, 1994), 57.

2. Bertrand Russell, *The Conquest of Happiness* (New York: W. W. Norton, 1996),
62.

Chapter 8

1. "By the Numbers Archive: Do You Ever Fantasize about Someone Else During
Sex?," Menstuff.org, accessed February 10, 2017, http://www.menstuff.org/
columns/numbers/archive.html.

Chapter 9

1. *Henry IV: Part II*, ed. Henry Hudson (Boston: Ginn, 1888), act 2, sc. 3.

2. J. Abram McBride, Culley C. Carson III, and Robert M Coward, "Testosterone Deficiency in the Aging Male," *Therapeutic Advances in Urology* 9, no. 1
(February 2016): 47–60.

Chapter 10

1. National Center for HIV/AIDS, Viral Hepatitis, STD, and TB Prevention, "Reported STDs in the United States: 2015 National Data for Chlamydia, Gonorrhea, and Syphilis," Centers for Disease Control and Prevention, October 2016, http://www.cdc.gov/nchhstp/newsroom/docs/factsheets/std-trends-508.pdf.

2. Centers for Disease Control and Prevention, "Chlamydia: CDC Fact Sheet (Detailed)," last modified October 17, 2016,

http://www.cdc.gov/std/chlamydia/stdfact-chlamydia-detailed.htm.

3. Centers for Disease Control and Prevention, "Tracking the Hidden Epidemics: Trends in STDs in the United States—Chlamydia," last reviewed January 5, 2016, https://wonder.cdc.gov/wonder/help/STD/Trends-Chlamydia.html.

4. Centers for Disease Control and Prevention, "Gonorrhea," last reviewed November 17, 2015 (archived), http://www.cdc.gov/std/stats12/gonorrhea.htm.

5. National Center for HIV/AIDS, Viral Hepatitis, STD, and TB Prevention, "Trends in Reportable Sexually Transmitted Diseases in the United States, 2005," Centers for Disease Control and Prevention, last reviewed December 13, 2006 (archived), http://www.cdc.gov/std/stats05/trends2005.htm.

6. National Center for HIV/AIDS, Viral Hepatitis, STD, and TB Prevention, "Reported Cases of STDs on the Rise in the U.S.," Centers for Disease Control and Prevention, last modified November 17, 2015, http://www.cdc.gov/nchhstp/newsroom/2015/std-surveillance-report-press-release.html.

7. Centers for Disease Control and Prevention, "Genital HSV Infections," last updated June 8, 2015, http://www.cdc.gov/std/tg2015/herpes.htm.

8. Centers for Disease Control and Prevention, "Genital HPV Infection: Fact Sheet," last modified January 3, 2017, http://www.cdc.gov/std/HPV/STD-Fact-HPV.htm#a7.

9. Centers for Disease Control and Prevention, "National Human Papillomavirus Vaccination Coverage among Adolescents Aged 13–17 Years — National Immunization Survey—Teen, United States, 2011," *Morbidity and Mortality Weekly Report* 63, no. 2 (September 2014): 61-70.

10. National Center for HIV/AIDS, Viral Hepatitis, STD, and TB Prevention, "HIV/AIDS Prevention," Centers for Disease Control and Prevention, last

modified December 21, 2016, http://www.cdc.gov/hiv/basics/prevention.html.

Chapter 12

1. Teri D. Fisher, Zachary T. Moore, and Mary-Jo Pittenger, "Sex on the Brain? An Examination of Frequency of Sexual Cognitions as a Function of Gender, Erotophilia, and Social Desirability," *Journal of Sex Research* 49, no. 1 (2012): 69–77, doi:10.1080/00224499.2011.565429.

2. "Male Circumcision and Risk for HIV Transmission and Other Health Conditions: Implications for the United States," Centers for Disease Control and Prevention, last modified February 2008, http://stacks.cdc.gov/view/cdc/13545; and World Health Organization, "Male Circumcision for HIV Prevention," http://www.who.int/hiv/topics/malecircumcision/en/.

3. American Cancer Society, *Cancer Facts & Figures: 2017* (Atlanta: American Cancer Society, 2017).

4. American Cancer Society, "Prostate Cancer Risk Factors," last modified March 11, 2016, http://www.cancer.org/cancer/prostatecancer/detailedguide/prostate-cancer-risk-factors.

5. Richard P. Gallagher and Neil Fleshner, "Prostate Cancer: Individual Risk Factors," *Canadian Medical Association Journal* 159 (October 6, 1998) 807–813, http://www.cmaj.ca/cgi/reprint/159/7/807.pdf.

6. American Cancer Society, "Testicular Cancer," January 2016, http://www.cancer.org/acs/groups/content/@nho/documents/document/testicularcancerpdf.pdf.

Chapter 14

1. Erick Janssen and John Bancroft, "The Dual Control Model: The Role of Sexual Inhibition and Excitation in Sexual Arousal and Behavior," in *The Psychopathology of Sex*, ed. Erick Janssen (Bloomington: Indiana University Press, 2007).

Index

A

abstinence, 50, 154, 174
abusive relationships, 145
addiction issues, 53, 152–153
adolescents/teens, 112, 123
   information given to, 7
   learning superpotency, 160–161
   masturbation, 199
   self-doubt, 13
aesthetics of genitals, 20–21
age/aging
   agelessness, 124–135
   andropause versus menopause, 131–132
   arteriosclerosis, 132–133
   birth to adolescence, 123
   changes in desire, 121–122
   current research on sex lives and, 133
   effects on orgasms, 156–157
   effects on sexual function, 9
   nocturnal erections and, 43
   premature ejaculation and, 55
   refractory period and, 38
   semen production and, 36
   young adulthood, 124
   young-at-heart attitude, 130–131
aggressive partners, 116
AIDS, 16, 103–104, 110, 139–140, 158
alcoholism, 53–54

alcohol use, 11, 53. *See also* recreational drug use
alprostadil (prostaglandin-E1 or PGE-1), 47, 79–81
alternative treatments for erectile dysfunction, 88–89
amphetamine use, 54
anabolic steroids, 49
anal cancer, 138–139
anal sex, 110, 140
anatomy
   male genitalia, 29–30, 34–36
   normal testicles, 164
   penis, 150–151
   urinary meatus, 20
androgen, 63, 127–128
andropause, 49, 128, 131–132
anger, 117–119
angina, 152
anxiety. *See also* performance anxiety
   common men's, 8
   dealing with, 99–100
   handling, 187–188
   physiological effects, 11
   premature ejaculation and, 57
aphrodisiacs, 31–32, 88–89
appearance of genitals, 20–21
arousal
   factors in, 30–32
   oral contact, 31
   in response to smells, 31–32

arousal (*continued*)
  in response to sounds, 32
  size of penis during, 27
  study on, 186–187
  with use of erectile dysfunction
      drugs, 74
  women's, 25
arterial insufficiency, 46
arteriography, penile, 46
arteriosclerosis, 48, 132
attitude, 72
  adjusting, 10
  superpotent, 72, 73, 93, 159,
      161
  winner, 180
Avodart (dutasteride), 63–64

B
Bacillus Calmette-Guérin (BCG), 162
Barnard, Christiaan, 88–89
behavior, men's, 168
  connection between penis and, 5
  making changes to, 10
benign prostate hypertrophy (BPH)
  description/overview, 61–63
  medical treatments, 63–64
  nonsurgical treatments (TUMT
      or DOT), 64
  prostatectomy, 63
  transurethral prostatectomy
      (TURP), 65–66
Bennis, Warren, 93–94
birth control, 153–154. *See also*
  condoms
bisexual men, 78
bladder cancer, 161–162
blood flow problems, 83

boredom, 108–109
BPH. *See* benign prostate
  hypertrophy (BPH)
bulbocavernosus reflex test, 45

C
CAD (coronary artery disease), 152
cancer
  anal, 139
  bladder, 161–162
  nonsurgical treatments, 69–70,
      161–162
  of penis, 158
  prostate, 66–70, 158–159,
      162–163
  testicular, 71, 164
cardiovascular disease, 46
cardiovascular fitness, 194
casual sex, 13
Caverject, 79–80
celebrities, sex appeal of, 178
Centers for Disease Control and
    Prevention (CDC)
  HIV/AIDS, 139–140
  sexually transmitted diseases,
      135
central nervous system, 53–54
character of superpotent men
  being a winner, 180
  being well-rounded, 181
  courage, 180
  expressing full potential, 180
  happiness, 181
  quality relationships, 181
  self-confidence, 179
chlamydia, 135–136
Cialis, 74, 78

circulatory problems, 47
circumcision, 157–158
the clap (gonorrhea), 136–137
claudication, 46
climax. *See* ejaculation; orgasms
cocaine use, 54
cock rings, 154–155
coming. *See* ejaculation
commonalities among men, 3–4
communication
    for achieving mutual
        satisfaction, 12
    advice for women, 142–143, 145
    about aversions, 146
    about conflicts, 117–119
    about feelings/expectations, 116
    importance of open/honest,
        192–193
    improving skills, 206
    for intimacy, 114–115
    about needs and desires, 150,
        156
    poor, 56
    about sex during sex, 186
    about use of medications for
        erectile dysfunction, 75–76
    value of, 75, 127
complaints, women's. *See* women's
    complaints
compulsive sexual activity, 152–
    153
condoms, 58, 110, 140, 154
confidence in penis and sexual
    performance, 5–6
constricting devices, 87–88
contagious diseases. *See* sexually
    transmitted diseases (STDs)

continence, after prostate surgery,
    67–68
control of ejaculation, 198–200
Coolidge effect, 105–106
coronary artery disease (CAD), 77,
    152
corpora cavernosa, 27, 30–33
corpus spongiosum, 29–30
courage, 180
Cowper's gland/Cowper's fluid, 35
cultural perceptions of vaginas and
    penises, 20–21
curiosity, women's, 8–9

D
damaging the penis, 150–151
Danoff's law, 147
dapoxetine (Priligy), 58
deformities of the penis,
    hypospadias, 20
delaying ejaculation, 58, 59,
    154–155, 201–203
demanding lovers, 116
depression, 52, 101–102, 187
desire. *See* sex drive (libido)
detumescence/tumescence, 32–33,
    43–44
diabetes, 47–48
diet/weight control, 194–195
differences among penises, 21
digital rectal examination (DRE),
    62, 68, 162
discharge, penile, 136
diseases. *See* medical causes of
    erectile dysfunction; sexually
    transmitted diseases (STDs)

dose-optimized thermal (DOT)
    therapy, 64
DRE (digital rectal examination),
    62, 68, 162
drugs. *See* alcohol use; medications
    (for erectile dysfunction);
    medications (in general);
    recreational drug use
dutasteride (Avodart), 63–64
dysfunction, sexual. *See* erectile
    dysfunction/impotence; sexual
    function (men)

E
Edex, 79–80
ego shapers, 6
ejaculation. *See also* semen/seminal
    fluid
    anxiety about, 9
    changes with age, 126–127,
        156–157
    concerns about, 39
    controlling timing, 198–200
    delayed, 127, 198–199
    delaying, 58, 59, 154–155,
        201–203
    effects of many, 151
    effects of medications on, 51–53
    influences on, 36
    lack of ability for, 198
    misinformation about, 13
    orgasm without, 34
    physiology of, 33, 35–36, 56–57
    premature (*See* premature
        ejaculation (PE))
    refractory period following,
        37–38

ejaculation (*continued*)
    retarded, 52
    retrograde, 66
    spontaneous, 198
    taint exercises, 200–201
    triggering of, 35–37
ejaculatory control, 198–200
ejaculatory reflex, 34, 35–36, 57,
    124, 199, 201
embarrassment, 8, 94–95
emergencies, priapism, 82
EMLA cream, 55
emotional issues. *See also* mental
    health issues
    handling negative emotions,
        187–188
    use of erectile dysfunction
        medications, 81
emotions, arousal and, 32
empowerment, 16–17
enlarged prostate, 63–65, 162
enlarging the penis, 150
enthusiasm, 114–115
environment/location, 112–113
erectile devices, 73, 87–88. *See also*
    penile implants/prostheses
erectile dysfunction/impotence, 7
    after prostatectomy, 67, 158–
        159
    alternative treatments, 88–89
    arteriosclerosis and, 132
    benefits of oral sex, 111
    compared to premature
        ejaculation, 56–57
    data on, 76
    definition, 9
    drugs for, 26–27

erectile dysfunction/impotence
(*continued*)
medical conditions (*see*
medical causes of erectile
dysfunction)
men's reluctance to talk about,
40–41
partial loss of erection, 88
physiological causes, 9
psychological factors in, 10 (*see
also* performance anxiety)
sexual enhancement products, 6
treatment (*see* treatment for
erectile dysfunction)
use of performance-enhancing
drugs without, 74
erections. *See also* tumescence/
detumescence
after prostate surgery, 67–68
anxiety about, 9
average size/length of, 22–23
changes with aging, 125
cocaine use and, 54
corpora cavernosa function, 27
effects of many, 151
effects of medications on,
51–53, 52
effects of sucking, 31
hardness of, 24
loss of, 47
mechanisms of, 123
nicotine and, 54–55
pharmacological, 80 (*see also*
medications (for erectile
dysfunction))
physical and emotional factors,
30–32

erections (*continued*)
physiology of, 29–30, 32–33
priapism, 80, 82
response to touch for, 31
during sleep, 42–43
smoking tobacco and, 54–55
erotic touch, 31
erotic videos, 186–187
estrogen, 131–132
exercise, 50, 100, 194, 196
exercises for superpotency
controlling your timing, 198–
200
pelvic control, 196–198
expectations
of older couples, 132
about sexual satisfaction, 12
unrealistic, 11, 116, 203

F
failure, penis. *See* erectile
dysfunction/impotence
fantasies, 106–107
fatigue, 109
fear of failure. *See* performance
anxiety
fears, rational/irrational, 103–104
females. *See* women
fertility, 49, 66, 136
finasteride (Proscar), 63
fitness/health, 193–196
flaccid penis, 22–23, 37
foreplay, 75, 111, 126, 144, 146,
155, 192
foreskin, 157–158
functions of penis, 29

G

Gardasil, 138, 139
gay community. *See* homosexual
    men
genital herpes, 138
genitals
    appearance/aesthetics of, 20–21
    male anatomy, 29–30
    preventing medical problems in,
        162–164
gonorrhea (the clap), 136–137

H

Hamilton, Scott, 71
happiness, 181
hard dick syndrome, 107–109
hardness of penis, 24
hard on demand myth, 109–110,
    116
HBP (high blood pressure), 46, 52
health/fitness, 193–196
heart disease, 151–152
herpes, genital, 138
high blood pressure (HBP), 46, 52
high intensity focused
    ultrasonography (HIFU),
        69–70
HIV/AIDS, 16, 103–104, 110, 136,
    137, 139–140, 158
HIV medications, 78–79
homosexual men, 78
    anal cancer, 139
    sexually transmitted diseases,
        138–139
hormonal causes of erectile
    dysfunction, 47–49
hostility toward partners, 117–119

HPV (human papillomavirus),
    138–139
human papillomavirus (HPV),
    138–139
humor, 97, 181
hygiene, 113–114, 158
hypersensitivity, 124
hypogonadism (testicular failure),
    48–49, 127–128
hypospadias, 20

I

idealization of sex act, 14–15
identity, sexual, 168
ignorance, about penis and
    sexuality, 6–8
illness. *See* medical causes of
    erectile dysfunction
imagination, arousal and, 32
immunotherapy, 162
implants. *See* penile implants/
    prostheses
impotence. *See* erectile
    dysfunction/impotence
inadequacy, 13, 116
incompatibility, 115
infectious diseases. *See* sexually
    transmitted diseases (STDs)
infertility, 136
inflatable prostheses, 84–85
inhibitory mechanisms, 54
injuries to penis, 150–151
insecurity
    embarrassing sexual experiences
        and, 6
    sexual/sensual aids and, 12
    size of penis, 25–26

inserting objects in penises, 151
intimidation, 115–117, 153

J
Johnson, Magic, 139
jokes, penis-related, 4

K
kidney failure, 71–72
King Penis, 5
Kinsey, Alfred, 30

L
laser ablation therapy, 65
learning about sex, 193
leg pain, 46
leisure world syndrome, 132–133
length of penis, 22–23
Levitra, 74
libido. *See* sex drive (libido)
life stages. *See* age/aging
location/environment, 112–113
low threshold of excitement,
     199–200
lubrication, 35, 40, 132, 145, 151,
     192, 199–200

M
macho posturing, 13–14
magnetic resonance imaging (MRI),
     68
male genitalia, 29–30, 34–35,
     35–36
male menopause, 127
malleable implants, 84–85
marijuana use, 54
masculinity, self-doubt about, 14
Masters and Johnson method, 59

masturbation, 51, 157, 198
mechanical erectile devices, 73,
     87–88
media
     effects on self-image, 14, 195
     hype about erectile dysfunction
          medications, 78
medical causes of erectile
     dysfunction, 39. *See also*
     urologic diseases/conditions
     causes of impotence, 40–44
     diagnostic tests, 43–44, 45, 46,
          51–52, 62, 66, 68
     hormonal, 47–49
     illness, 49–51
     injectable drugs for diagnosis
          and treatment, 47
     neurological disorders, 45
     prescribed medications, 51–53
     ruling out correctable, 85
     steroid use, 49
     vascular disorders, 45–46
medications (for erectile
     dysfunction), 26–27, 47, 74–75
     for benign prostate hypertrophy,
          63–64
     candidates for, 132–133
     cautions for using, 75–76, 81,
          152
     crutch effect of, 93
     for delaying ejaculation, 58, 59
     dosages, 77, 80–83
     effectiveness of, 76–77
     hype about, 78
     injectable, 77, 80–83
     Muse system, 77, 79–80
     for premature ejaculation, 55

medications (*continued*)
    recreational use of, 78
    selective serotonin reuptake
        inhibitors (SSRIs), 58
    side effects of, 77, 80, 82
    transdermal applications, 130
    using combinations of, 82
medications (in general)
    effects on sexual function, 11,
        51–53
    HIV medications with PDE-5
        inhibitors, 78–79
    prescription, 51–53
menopause, 131–132
mental health issues, 195–196. *See
    also* anxiety; emotional issues;
    performance anxiety
    depression, 52, 101–102, 187
    psychological impotence, 43–44,
        198
micropenises, 149
microwave therapy, 64
mind-altering substances, 54
misconceptions/misinformation, 6,
    29–30. *See also* myths
moral obligations, 184–185,
    185–186
morning sex, 109–110
morning wood, 43–44, 110
MRI (magnetic resonance imaging),
    68
mumps, 48
Muse system, 77, 79–80
mutual masturbation, 51
myths
    hard on demand, 109–110, 116
    heart damage from sex, 151–152

myths (*continued*)
    penile enhancement procedures,
        26–28
    penis-related, 6
    size of penis, 21–22
    wearing out your penis, 16

N
narcotics, 54–55
National Institutes of Health
    (NIH), 76
needs, men's, 150, 155–156, 193
negative penis personalities,
    172–175
negative thinking, 99–100, 203–
    204
Neo-Synephrine, 82
neurological causes of erectile
    dysfunction, 45, 48, 53–54
neurovascular bundle, 67
nicknames, for penises, 4–5
nicotine, 54–55
NIH (National Institutes of
    Health), 76
nocturnal erections, 42–44
nocturnal penile tumescence (NPT)
    test, 43–44
nonsexual erections, 123
normal penis, 9
NPT (nocturnal penile tumescence)
    test, 43–44

O
objects in penises, 151
obsessive sexual activity, 152–153
obstructions, prostatic. *See* benign
    prostate hypertrophy (BPH)

odors, 113–114
older adulthood, 126–127
oral contact, men's response to, 31
oral sex, 51, 110, 140
orchitis, 48
organic impotence, 43, 44, 45, 89
orgasms
    anxiety about, 9
    changes with age, 125–127
    definition/description, 33–34
    effects of aging, 156–157
    effects of many, 151
    physiology of, 57
    prolonging, 157
    size of penis and, 24–25

P
Pampered Penis Personality, 175
partial loss of erection, 88
Passionate Penis Personality, 170
Paxil, 58
PDE-5 inhibitors, 58, 59, 74
PE. See premature ejaculation (PE)
Pedestrian Penis Personality, 174
penetration, ability for, 9
penile arteriography, 46
penile enhancement procedures,
    26–28
penile implants/prostheses, 24, 73,
    84–86
    bad candidates for, 86–87
    good candidates for, 132–133
    cautions/contraindications, 88
    ideal candidates, 86, 87
    mechanical devices, 87–88
penis
    anatomy, 29–30

penis (continued)
    cancer of, 158
    changes through life stages, 123
    response to touch, 30
penis awareness, 183
penis enlargement, 150
penis envy, 8–9
penis mystique, 7–8
penis orientation, 4–6, 182, 205
Penis Paradox, 98–99, 100, 108,
    125
penis personalities, 167–168, 176
    Pampered Penis Personality, 175
    Passionate Penis Personality,
        170
    Pedestrian Penis Personality,
        174
    Pensive Penis Personality, 170
    Perceptive Penis Personality, 169
    Pious Penis Personality, 174
    Pipe-Dream Penis Personality,
        173
    Poetic Penis Personality, 171
    Pompous Penis Personality, 173
    Possessive Penis Personality, 175
    Procrastinating Penis
        Personality, 172
    Prodigious Penis Personality,
        172
    Psychedelic Penis Personality,
        171
    Purposeful Penis Personality,
        169
penis power. See also superpotent
    men
    changes with age, 121–122 (see
        also age/aging)

penis power (*continued*)
 discovering, 177–179, 188–189
 educating sons about, 147–148
 effect of circumcision on, 158
 exercises for, 196–201
 foundations of, 179
 after kidney transplants, 71–72
 loss after prostate surgery, 69
 meaning of, 205–206
 medical conditions affecting
  (*see* erectile dysfunction/
  impotence; medical causes
  of erectile dysfunction)
 positive penis personalities,
  169–172
 secret of, 16–17
 summer increase of, 156
 after vasectomy, 154

penis weakness
 negative feedback loop, 187
 negative penis personalities,
  172–175
 reasons for current epidemic,
  11–15
 ruling out medical problems (*see*
  medical causes of erectile
  dysfunction)
 sudden onset, 164
 truths and myths about, 8–10
 in young men, 124
penocentricity, 4
Pensive Penis Personality, 170
Perceptive Penis Personality, 169
performance, 15, 49, 203–204
performance anxiety, 117, 186–187
 acknowledging, 96–99

performance anxiety (*continued*)
 depression with, 101–102
 descriptions, causes, 91–92
 guilt as factor in, 102–103
 medical solutions, 92–93
 positive thinking, 94–96
 superpotency, 99–101
 Wallenda factor, 93–94
perineal contractions, 37
perineum, 198–200
personalities, penis. *See* penis
 personalities
PGE-1 (prostaglandin-E1 or
 alprostadil), 47, 79–81
phalloplasty, 26–28, 150
pheromones, 31–32
physicians
 common questions asked by
  patients, 7–8
 discussions of sexuality by, 6
physiology
 ejaculation, 33, 35–36, 56–57
 erections, 29–30, 32–33
 male sex act, 34–35
 response to oral sex, 111
 sexuality, 74–75
 size of penis, 25
 stress response, 11
"the pills," 73–74. *See also*
 treatment for erectile
 dysfunction
Pious Penis Personality, 174
Pipe-Dream Penis Personality, 173
piss hard-ons, 43–44
pleasure
 caring about partner's, 186
 giving and receiving, 184

pleasure (*continued*)
  mutual, 185
pleasure response, 36–37. *See also*
  ejaculation; orgasms
Poetic Penis Personality, 171
Pompous Penis Personality, 173
positive penis personalities,
  169–172
Possessive Penis Personality, 175
postage stamp test, 44
potency, 23–25
potential of superpotent men, 180
premature ejaculation (PE), 13, 39,
  124
  description and definitions,
    55–56, 199
  getting help, 56–57
  history of treating, 59
  low threshold of excitement,
    199–200
  off-label prescription
    medications, 58, 59
  self-help approaches, 58
prescription medications, 51–53
priapism, 80, 82, 154
Priligy (dapoxetine), 58
Procrastinating Penis Personality,
  172
Prodigious Penis Personality, 172
progressive testosterone deficiency,
  127–128
prolactin, 48
prolonging orgasms, 157
Promescent, 55
Proscar (finasteride), 63
prostaglandin-E1 (PGE-1 or
  alprostadil), 47, 79–81

prostate, 34, 35. *See also* benign
  prostate hypertrophy (BPH)
  enlarged, 63–65, 162
  preventing diseases of, 163–164
prostate cancer, 66–70, 158–159,
  162–163
prostatectomy, 63–64
prostheses, penile. *See* penile
  implants/prostheses
protease inhibitors, 78–79
Prozac, 58
Psychedelic Penis Personality, 171
psychological impotence, 43–44,
  198. *See also* performance
  anxiety
puberty, 123
Purposeful Penis Personality, 169

Q
quality of life, 56, 67
questions asked by patients, 7–8

R
radiation therapy, 69
reality/truths
  about penises, 17
  sexual, 14–15
  size of penis (*see* size of penis)
recreational drug use, 53–54. *See
  also* alcohol use
reflexes, 45
  bulbocavernosus reflex test, 45
  contraction of scrotum, 37
  ejaculatory, 34, 35–36, 57, 124,
    199, 201
  gag, 111

refractory period, 37–38, 57, 106,
    124, 125–126
relationships
    abusive, 145
    having quality, 181
    making friends with your penis,
        204–205
    problems in, 117–119
    rifts in, 147
    symbiotic, with penis, 182
religious issues, 102–103
resentment, 118
retarded ejaculation, 39, 198
retrograde ejaculation, 66
risks of testosterone replacement
    therapy, 128–130
role modeling for sons, 159–161
roles of penis, 29
routineness of sex, 107–109,
    109–110
Russell, Bertrand, 100

S

satisfaction
    factors in, 37
    incompatibility issues, 115
    mutual, 187
    of partner, 203
    with sex life, 183–184
    size of penis and, 25
scrotum, 37, 156
secret of penis power, 16–17
selective serotonin reuptake
    inhibitors (SSRIs), 58
self-confidence, 179

self-doubt
    causes/creation of, 14, 143, 157,
        159
    effects of, 6, 14, 98, 124, 188,
        198
    elimination of, 16, 21, 203–204
    lack of, 14
    triggers of, 116
    vicious cycle of, 10, 13
    vulnerability to, 106
    about your masculinity, 95–96,
        195
self-education, 191–193
self-esteem, 14, 95–96, 97–98, 112
self-examination of testicles, 164
self-interest, 192
self-perception, penis size and, 5
semen/seminal fluid, 34–35, 36, 38
    change in volume of, 156–157
    swallowing, 145–146
seminal vesicles, 34, 38
senses, arousal responses to, 31–32
sensitivity to touch, 37
sensual aids, vibrators, 12
setbacks, 93, 112
sex act
    effect of odors, 113–114
    enjoyment/lack of enjoyment,
        15–16
    fear of failure, 94
    media-related idealization of,
        14–15
    medical reasons for adapting/
        limiting, 50–51
    as performance, 203–204
    unpleasant aspects of, 114–115
sex appeal, 178

sex drive (libido), 49
    changes through life stages, 123,
        125–126
    differences between partners,
        155–156
    diminished, 39, 48
    effects of medications on, 63–64
    kidney disease and, 71–72
    levels of desire, 153
    loss of, 9, 101–102, 155
    postmenopausal women, 132
    reasons for diminished, 52
    recreational drug use and, 53–55
    use of erectile dysfunction drugs
        without, 74–75
sex life
    after kidney transplants, 71–72
    age and, 87, 126, 133
    emotional issues, 112
    improving, 111
    inhibitors, 103
    invigorating your, 109
    physical problems and, 162
    satisfaction with your, 57
    self-esteem and, 96
    sense of adventure, 108
    sexual ignorance and, 142
    of superpotent men, 183–184
    use of pills, 76
sex objects, 185–186
sexual activity
    compulsive/obsessive, 152–153
    environment/location, 112–113
    frequency of, 150–151, 199
    with heart disease, 151–152
    for preventing prostate
        problems, 163–164

sexual enhancement products, 6,
    11, 12. *See also* medications
    (for erectile dysfunction)
sexual frustration, 16
sexual function (men)
    abnormal (*see* erectile
        dysfunction/impotence)
    categories of dysfunction, 39
    effects of medications on, 51–53
    effects of stress on, 11
    normal, 10
    size of penis and, 23–24
sexual function (women), 11–12
sexual identity, 168
sexuality
    discussions with doctors, 7
    ease with, 185–186
    as fundamental human drive, 6
    ignorance about, 6–8
    lack of information, 12–13
    limiting your, 50
    physiology of, 74–75
    standards of, 13
    "the talk," 7
sexually transmitted diseases
    (STDs), 78. *See also* condoms
    chlamydia, 135–136
    genital herpes, 138
    gonorrhea (the clap), 136–137
    HIV/AIDS, 103–104, 110, 135,
        136, 137, 139–140
    human papillomavirus (HPV),
        138–139
    syphilis, 137
    transmission of, 110
sexual response phases, 57

size of penis
  chubby versus thin men, 26
  clichés about, 24
  micropenises, 149
  myth of importance of, 25–26
  physiology and satisfaction
      related to, 25
  potency and, 23–25
  preoccupation with, 21–22
  problems with large, 145
  thinking small versus big, 26
  truth about, 19
  variations in, 22–23
  women's preferences, 149–150
sleep, erections during, 42–44
smell, arousal response to, 31–32
smoking, 54–55
sounds, erotic impact of, 32
sperm, 34, 35, 36
squeeze technique, 59, 202–203
SSRIs (selective serotonin reuptake
    inhibitors), 58–59
SST deformity, 85–86
standards
  adolescent, 13
  living up to, 195
  men's self-imposed, 15
  mythological, 10
  setting your own, 96
  of sexuality, 13
Staxyn, 74
staying power, 57
STDs. See sexually transmitted
    diseases (STDs)
Stendra, 74

stimulation
  enhancement of medications
      with, 81
  methods, 25
  pharmacologic erections and, 77
  physiological effects of, 30
  premature ejaculation with, 56
  reflex action of ejaculation, 35
  during refractory period, 37
  visual, 32
stop-start technique, 59
stress, 11, 101, 187–188, 195–196
superpotent men, 12, 52, 65,
    99–101, 131, 156. See also
    penis power
  age issues, 130–132
  attitude of superpotency, 72, 73,
      93, 161
  avoiding negative thinking/self-
      doubt, 203–204
  being a role model, 148, 159–
      161
  cardiovascular fitness, 194
  character of, 179–181
  controlling timing, 198–200
  definition, 17
  diet/weight control, 194–195
  discovering penis power,
      177–179, 188–189
  ease with sexuality, 185–186
  enjoyment of variety, 184–185
  examples of, 117, 122
  finding your penis personality,
      167–176
  fulfilling sexual needs, 155–156
  getting rest, 195
  getting/staying fit, 193

superpotent men (*continued*)
  giving/receiving pleasure, 184
  giving without reservation, 186
  handling stress, 187–188
  intimidation by women, 116
  living up to standards, 195
  masturbation and, 157
  mental health, 195–196
  pelvic control, 196–198
  penis awareness, 183
  penis failure, 143
  performance anxiety, 186–187
  preferences of, 104
  and premature ejaculation, 59
  prosthetic implants and, 86
  role modeling for sons, 159–161
  satisfaction with sex life,
    183–184
  self-education, 191–193
  sexually transmitted diseases
    and, 104, 138–139
  skills for being, 99–100
  symbiotic relationship with
    penis, 182
  women's attitudes toward, 78,
    142
surgical procedures
  enlarging the penis, 150
  for penile enhancement/
    enlargement, 26–27
  penile implants/prostheses, 24,
    73, 84–86
  penis transplants, 83
  prostatectomy, 63–64, 159
  vasectomies, 153–154
symbiotic relationship with your
  penis, 182

syphilis, 137

T

taint exercises, 200–201
taste, erotic response to, 32
testicles, 34, 37
  injuries/illnesses of, 48
  self-examination, 164
  small, 49
testicular cancer, 71, 164
testicular failure (hypogonadism),
  48–49
testosterone, 125
  cautions for use of, 49
  deficiency of, 48
  low levels of, 39
  after removal of testes, 71
  sexual capacity with, 153
testosterone replacement therapy
  (TRT), 127–130
thermal therapy, 64
"the talk," 7
thyroid conditions, 48
tobacco use, 54–55
touch, sensitivity to, 37
transurethral microwave therapy
  (TUMT), 64
transurethral prostatectomy
  (TURP), 65–66
transurethral resection of bladder
  tumor (TURBT), 161
treatment for erectile dysfunction,
  73–74
  history of, 73–74
  PDE-5 inhibitors, 58, 59, 74
  vacuum erectile device (VED), 73
  Viagra, 11, 58, 73

TRT (testosterone replacement
    therapy), 127–130
truth. *See* reality/truths
tumescence/detumescence, 32–33,
    43–44
TUMT (transurethral microwave
    therapy), 64
tunica, 30
TURBT (transurethral resection of
    bladder), 161
TURP (transurethral
    prostatectomy), 65–66

U

unresponsive partners, 114–115
urethra, 29–30, 36
urinary meatus, 20
urination, 35
    benign prostate hypertrophy
        and, 61–62
    morning erections and, 43–44
    painful/burning, 163
urine, 29, 35
    blood in, 161
urologic diseases/conditions
    benign prostate hypertrophy
        (BPH), 61–66
    bladder cancer, 161–162
    kidney failure, 71–72
    preventing, 162–164
    prognosis and outlook, 71–72
    prostate cancer, 66–70
    symptoms, 162–163

V

vacuum erectile devices (VEDs), 73,
    87–88

vaginas, cultural perceptions of, 20
Valsalva maneuver, 203
vascular causes of erectile
    dysfunction, 45–46
    drugs for diagnosing and
        treating, 47
vasectomies, 153–154
venous leaks, 47, 83
Venus envy, 157
Viagra, 11, 58, 73, 74, 92–93
vibrators, 12
virility enhancers, 88–89
visual stimulation, erotic response
    to, 32

W

Wallenda, Karl, 93–94
Wallenda factor, 93–94
weight control, 194–195
well-roundedness, 181
winner attitude, 180
women
    advice for, 141–142, 205
    attitudes toward oral sex, 111
    cautions for anal sex with, 110
    communication by/with,
        142–143
    effects of EMLA on, 55
    gonorrhea in, 137
    human papillomavirus (HPV),
        138–139
    hygiene issues, 113–114
    infertility causes, 136
    interest in penis size, 23–24
    interest in superpotency, 78
    menopause, 131–132
    penis orientation by, 148

women (*continued*)
    penis preferences, 149–150
    postnatal changes, 155
    understanding differences, 192
women's complaints
    alcohol use by partner, 147
    distasteful demands, 145–146
    educating sons about penis
        power, 147–148
    getting turned down for sex, 144
    men's businesslike approach to
        sex, 144
    men's discomfort with touch,
        146–147
    not being in the mood, 143
    pain during sex, 144–145
    relationship rifts, 147
    unimaginative sex, 146
women's movement, 11–12
women's sexuality, 6–8

Y
yohimbine therapy, 88–89

Z
Zoloft, 58

About the Author

Dudley Seth Danoff, MD, FACS, is a diplomate of the American Board of Urology and a fellow of the American College of Surgeons. Born in Brooklyn, New York, Dr. Danoff is a graduate of Princeton University, summa cum laude and Phi Beta Kappa. He received his medical degree at Yale University with honors. He completed his urologic surgical training and fellowship at Columbia University Presbyterian Medical Center in New York City. Following his training, he served as a major in the United States Air Force Medical Corps. For more than a quarter century, Dr. Danoff taught on the clinical faculty of UCLA School of Medicine. Currently, he is attending urologic surgeon at Cedars-Sinai Medical Center in Los Angeles. He is the founder and president of the prestigious Cedars-Sinai Medical Center Tower Urology Medical Group, the leading urologic practice serving the Southern California community for over thirty years. Dr. Danoff and his wife, Israeli singer Hedva Amrani, are longtime residents of Beverly Hills, California, and have two children: Aurele Danoff, an attorney, and Doran Danoff, a composer.

Dr. Danoff invites you to stay in touch:

Facebook: https://www.facebook.com/TheUltimateGuidetoMaleHealth/
Twitter: https://twitter.com/DrDanoff
LinkedIn: http://bit.ly/2qMcVr8
Website: http://theultimateguidetomenshealth.com/
Blog: http://theultimateguidetomenshealth.com/blog/
E-mail: AskDrDanoff@theultimateguidetomenshealth.com